Managing Yourself

Titles in the series

Barbara Scammell: Communication Skills

Communication in society
The communications continuum: forms and skills
The communications continuum: coaching and counselling
Planning and organising
Staffing
Co-ordinating
Communication in nurse management at the point of service delivery
Communication in nurse management in different areas of medical care

Verena Tschudin with Jane Schober: Managing Yourself

'Know thyself'
Valuing yourself
Motivating yourself
Asserting yourself
Stressing yourself
Supporting yourself
Celebrating yourself
Your career – making the choices

Sheila Marson (ed.): Managing People

The science and function of management
Team building: a practical approach
Leadership
Creating a climate for learning
Quality and its control

Annabel Broome: Managing Change

Principles of complex change
Leadership and creating change from within
Imposed change
The nurse as a change agent
Identifying training and development needs
Appendix A: Health of the organisation questionnaire
Appendix B: Role effectiveness profile – tool for self-assessment

Diana Sale: Quality Assurance

An introduction to quality assurance
Standards of care
Quality assurance measures – performance. Nursing audit
Quality assurance measures – performance. Quality patient care scale
Quality assurance measures – performance. Monitor – an index of the
quality of nursing care
Quality circles
Measuring outcome standards – using a computerised nursing
system (Excelcare)

Financial Budgeting

(*in preparation*)

ESSENTIALS OF NURSING MANAGEMENT

Managing Yourself

Verena Tschudin

with Jane Schober

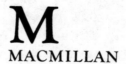

MACMILLAN

First published 1990 by
THE MACMILLAN PRESS LTD
Houndmills, Basingstoke, Hampshire RG21 2XS
and London
Companies and representatives
throughout the world

ISBN 0–333–48431–2

A catalogue record for this book is available
from the British Library.

Printed in Hong Kong

Reprinted 1991, 1992, 1993

Contents

Acknowledgements

The author would like to thank Jane Schober very particularly for writing the chapter on career choices; special thanks also to Margaret Wellings, for turning yet another set of scrap papers into a manuscript; and to Jill Baker, for helping and encouraging this project to completion.

The author and publishers would like to thank the following photographic sources:

Sally and Richard Greenhill

The Photo Co-op

Topham Picture Library

Preface

'Management' has become one of those magic words: as long as you manage you're OK.

Management usually means 'other people'. In this book it means yourself. And this is where the problem starts. We generally know how to manage others. We know what they should do, how they should behave, how they should do their job, look after their children, deal with their colleagues, and so on. But to apply these same principles to ourselves is not nearly as easy.

This book starts with the principle that 'charity begins at home'. This doesn't mean indulging ourselves in all sorts of excesses: it means on the contrary a kind of discipline which doesn't shrink away from looking at the good *and* bad in us, the strengths *and* weaknesses, the helpful *and* unhelpful, the possible *and* impossible parts of ourselves. This can sometimes be daunting. It is not easy to face up to the darker side of the reality that we are, or make choices which lead us into the unknown. But it is often there that discoveries are made which can and will transform our lives.

As a nurse you are first of all a *person*. And although addressed to you as a nurse, this book looks at you as a person behind the uniform. It is meant for you the person, to be more effective in your work as a nurse: to manage yourself and others better.

Verena Tschudin
January 1990

Prologue: The dream . . .

Last night I had a dream:

I was one of a team of three sisters in charge of a large surgical ward. It was very busy, with constant coming and going of patients, staff of every kind and managers of this and that. These managers always had clipboards and asked many questions, looking cool while they did their surveys.

Then came a call that a disaster had happened nearby, and all senior staff were needed there. I was among those who went, repeatedly crawling through rubble and fallen masonry to try and get to injured people. The more frantically we searched, the more people we found, some very badly injured. The destruction seemed to go on and on.

After a while I crawled up from some cellar, still in uniform, very dusty, my cap grey and not straight on my head. I was dazed and shaking, not able to say anything. I was looking for someone to talk to, but I knew nobody; they were all too busy, but many seemed to be running around 'doing' nothing in particular, and with frightened looks on their faces.

I sat down in all this rubble and chaos, now not caring any more about anyone else. Tears started to flow and they seemed to fall very heavily on my lap, having gathered a lot of dirt and grime off my cheeks. That seemed to attract a person who came up very quietly from somewhere. I recognised the person, but it was not someone I knew by name. She helped me up, took my arm, and we picked a way through the chaos to some big gate. We stood there a long time, looking at the devastation and also out to ordinary life, and gradually I began to feel 'me' again. I was longing for a wash and clean-up, and to get back to work, in a new uniform, and feeling in charge again.

Chapter 1   'Know thyself'

Awareness

'Know thyself' was apparently written over the entrance to the temple of Apollo at Delphi. The oracle situated there seemed normally to have given obscure responses. To 'know thyself' is a clear enough instruction, but one which becomes obscure in the application.

Nurses have a better idea of the intricate workings of the body than do most people. But nurses do not necessarily have a better understanding of the wider implications of these workings of the body than do other people. As a patient said, 'Cancer isn't only a physical thing, it's also an emotional thing; above all it's a spiritual thing' (Lefébure, 1985).

Getting to know yourself is not necessarily painful. It *can* be painful, but essentially it is liberating.

Henry

After a lot of searching Henry had decided that, at the age of 42, he had gone through life like a snail: slow, cumbersome, and retreating too often into his shell. It was a revelation to Henry when he recognised that, like a snail, he had also left a silvery train behind him: wherever he had passed, something precious of himself had remained.

Awareness and **self-discovery** are not ends in themselves. They are there to help you discover the wider meaning of life in general and your place in it in particular. They help you to get the maximum out of life.

We make an impact on life whether we like it or not. To know what that impact — that silvery line — is, we have actually to be *aware* what kind of mark we make, and where. We have to be aware — of the body, the emotions, the mind, the spirit, the environment. They shape us, but we shape them too.

All search for impact, for change, for success, starts here and now. No book can give you interpersonal skills: you have them already. But this book aims to help you to become aware of, and to improve and utilise your skills.

Awareness of the body

Most people criticise their bodies. Hair grows where it shouldn't; a muscle is too tight; a pain too limiting; the digestion too fast or too slow; the nails not as attractive as someone else's. In order to use our bodies effectively we need to co-operate with them rather than chastise them.

We influence our bodies with clothes, diet and exercise. But our bodies are also influenced by biorhythms; by the time of day, the environment, our lifestyle and our character.

Wherever you are, stop in the position you are. Notice the position of your body. Just notice it — don't change it.

- Are you comfortable? What is your position saying to you?
- What is your position saying about you to others?
- If you like, change your position to one more comfortable, significant, evocative . . .
- What would you most like to express at this moment with your body? Do it.

In order to learn more effective awareness of the body, try to:

- be aware without judging;

- acknowledge without criticising;
- accept without blaming.

When you are aware of your body, you are also aware of the space around it.

At a station . . .

The following took place at a tube station.

A very pretty girl with noisy shoes went up to a smallish middle-aged man wearing a cloth cap. In a loud voice she said, 'Hello, darling', then walked away. As a train pulled in she made her way to the man again, going close up but saying nothing. Hastily, he walked to another carriage. The girl stood outside, laughing loudly at him.

Do you know what your usual defence is when someone gets too close? Would you normally use words or body language to defend yourself? The interpretation we give of our own and other people's behaviour shapes our lives much more significantly than we are aware most of the time.

Awareness of the body is so basic that we tend to overlook its impact and take it for granted. The way we walk, talk, dress; what we eat and how; how we look at others and let them look at us: all these things matter. They say who we are, and we say to the world who and what we are — or what we think we are, or would like the world to think we are, or imagine that we are, or would like to be.

Awareness of the senses

The senses are the go-betweens between the outer world of the body and the inner world of the emotions, the mind, the psyche, the soul.

We often say 'I see' and this has nothing to do with the physical eyes and the sense of **seeing**, but with the 'inner eye', the perception.

When you meet a person you know in the street you *see* that person, but with your inner eyes you 'see' past meetings with that person, and this colours your behaviour now. When you see a plate of pasta you remember the last time you had a plate of pasta: on a holiday in Italy; with a friend; or because you didn't know what else to choose from the menu.

The physical senses are the parts of the person that locate you in the world, give meaning to your past and present, and shape your future. What happens in the outside world is interiorised by the senses in order to shape the personality.

The sense of **hearing** conveys a sound from the physical world to that of understanding and knowing. When you hear correctly you can respond correctly. And it is in responding that we are 'humanised'. We express ourselves most truly when we respond: to people, events, insights, dreams.

Stop for a moment and become aware of all the sounds around you. Listen to them. Does any one sound mean anything in particular? If so, stay with that sound and its meaning for as long as feels appropriate.

'Love goes through the stomach' is perhaps the best-known adage of the sense of **taste**. Whenever we celebrate something we do so with food or drink. What do you think is the significance of this?

Some people who are very ill lose their sense of taste, as do patients on certain treatments. There is a correlation between losing taste and losing zest for life.

Think of your favourite food for a moment, and be aware of the expression on your face, the flow of saliva and the flow of gastric juices. Be aware of what you are saying to and about yourself with this.

The sense of **smell** is closely linked to taste. If you could never smell that the food you are cooking is in fact burning, you would not enjoy eating it either!

Touching, the last sense, is extremely important for nurses. There is a difference between giving an injection and giving an injection that will help the patient to get better.

A touch can be comforting and can also be hurtful. It can be given with meaning, as when holding someone close; or it can be a holding on for dear life, when someone is frightened. A handshake will reveal cold, warm, sweaty, or trembling hands and in this way give a good indication of that person's state of health or mind.

The sense of touch is not only something sensual, but also something sensuous. The traditionally inhibited Britons are only too well aware of this! Touching, above all other senses, is surrounded by taboos. We have only to think of the fear of many nurses of caring for patients with AIDS. The patients themselves say that what is most significant to them is the reaching out to them in the form of touch. How, when and where do you touch a person who expresses a need to be touched?

Awareness of the environment

To be aware of the body means also to be aware of the environment. Without the earth's gravity we wouldn't be able to walk, and a person's first deed anywhere – in the kitchen, in the train, in the ward – is to make an impact on that environment, simply by walking into it.

The environment – the house you live in, the area you grew up in, the air you breathe, the newspaper you read, the way to work, the work you do, the places you go to for leisure – all these shape you and condition you to be the person you are. A patient who looks out on a park with a pond and flowers, who sees people picnicking and children playing, is likely to get better quicker than one whose view is a brick wall without even any sky.

It has been said that you are what you eat, or read. In the same way you are what you look out on; you are what surrounds you, the places you visit. 'Your house is your larger body' writes Gibran (1926).

Awareness of the environment may mean for one person the ability to have a clean house and place of work, and for another the ability to be totally absorbed in a sunrise; to live in a high-rise flat, or to join the women at Greenham Common. Nature and nurture have given us possibilities and values. In turn we take those values and by our lives shape the environment for ourselves and others.

Think for a moment:

● What aspect of the environment, near or far, makes a deep impression on you?
● What part of the environment have you yourself shaped?
● What part would you *like* to shape, or change, and how?

There are no right or wrong answers to such questions. What is right for you is the best, and only that matters. Simply taking note of something puts you in relation to it, and the relationship you have – the way you respond to her, him, or it – makes you the person you are.

Awareness of temperament

In order to manage ourselves well we need to know ourselves well. **Self-knowledge** develops as contacts with people develop. Differences become accentuated and preferences for acting in one way or another become clear.

There are many systems in use for defining people's temperaments and characteristics. Astrology is well known; Chinese horoscopes have become familiar in the West; and from olden times people have been labelled according to the four body-humours believed to exist: sanguine (blood), choleric (bile), melancholic (black bile) and phlegmatic (phlegm).

The psychologist C. G. Jung also found that people fell into four broad types: thinking, feeling, sensing and intuiting. These categories have been simplified and made accessible by Isabel Myers and her mother Katherine C. Briggs in what they call the **Myers–Briggs Type Indicator**. This is detailed below. However, if you are already familiar with another system and find that helpful, follow the system that you find most suitable.

The Myers-Briggs Type Indicator

As you read through this outline of the Myers–Briggs Type Indicator, try to see into which type you yourself fit most readily. The ideal would be that each of us would be capable of functioning equally well in all categories. The fact is that we have clear 'preferences', but with the equally clear possibility of developing the opposite, or **shadow**, quality.

Extraverted/introverted

The first distinction made in Myers–Briggs is the 'orientation': **extraversion (E)** or **introversion (I)**. The way to find out simply which you are is to ask yourself this question: do you get your energy from being with people, or from being alone?

Extravert people are sociable. They like to be with and around people and they get very lonely when they are not surrounded. They are the life and soul of a party because they need (for their energy) to be the centre of attraction.

Olive	Olive is 87 and housebound. She was a teacher and the writer of dozens of books for children. Now every day is the 'worst ever'. She complains that nobody bothers about her, and that everybody is rude to her. She feels utterly lonely, though every day she will have at least the visit of the district nurse, the home-help, a neighbour and the meals-on-wheels service. Radio and TV are uninteresting: anything where she is not the centre of attraction is boring.

Introvert (I) people, on the other hand, are very territorial. They need space around them, both physical space and mental space. They often pursue activities on their own as they recharge their batteries in this way. In a crowd they can feel very lonely and disconnected, and after half an hour at a party they are ready to go home. They often work well *with* people, but it strains them.

No one is totally either extraverted or introverted. Each needs the other, but the suppressed, or shadow, side is less obvious. In Western society about 75 per cent of the population are extraverted (Keirsey & Bates, 1984), which means that introverted people tend to have more difficulty in feeling accepted. To be told that it is 'OK' to be introverted can be a considerable relief for these people.

Sensing/intuitive

The main characteristics of the temperament are the 'functions': sensing and intuiting, thinking and feeling. Each person 'prefers' one of the functions in each pair.

To know, roughly, whether you are either a **sensing (S)** or **intuitive (N)** type – 'N' is used as 'I' already stands for introversion – ask yourself this: would you describe yourself mainly as a practical (S) or as an innovative (N) person? Do you prefer actualities (S) or possibilities (N)? It appears that sensing people constitute about 75 per cent of the population, and intuitives about 25 per cent (Keirsey & Bates, 1984).

Sensing people need things to be realistic. They trust experience, the past, down-to-earth facts, and actuality. They are also very good at picking up details. In short, they trust anything that their senses have experienced. Small wonder perhaps, that sensing people make good nurses, doctors and policemen.

Intuiting people on the other hand are often described by others as having their heads in the clouds. They like what is possible, in the future. They will accept change as a challenge, and are always interested in growth. While sensing persons see details, intuitives see wholes. They make connections, trust images and hunches, and enjoy metaphors and ideas. They are the inventors, innovators and pioneers, both in science and in the arts.

Briggs Myers (1980) believes that differences in national characteristics between the British and American can be described in terms of the differences between sensing and intuiting. The appeal of the New World drew the intuitives to the West like bees to honey, leaving a proportionally large share of sensing people in Britain to enjoy their afternoon tea, Beefeaters, and the long weekend!

Thinking/feeling

The next division is between **thinking** (T) and **feeling** (F). Here the division in the population is about half and half, though men tend to be the thinking, and women the feeling, types.

The simple question to ask yourself here is: do you prefer to make decisions based on personal impact (F), or on principle, logic or objectivity (T)?

Since the education system stresses all the aspects of thinking, people who are naturally feeling types often also have well-developed thinking capacities, whereas thinking types are less likely to have developed their feeling characteristics.

Thinking people like words such as 'objectivity', 'principle', 'law', 'justice', 'analysis', 'firmness'. To a *feeling* person's ear, words like 'values', 'persuasion', 'personal', 'humane', 'harmony', 'appreciation' and 'devotion' are music.

Feeling people will often label thinkers as cold, calculating, remote and heartless. Conversely, thinkers will label feeling people as emotional and illogical, and as wearing their hearts on their sleeves.

Both types of people experience feelings. The thinking types however tend not to show them, but instead internalise them (which may account for the fact that more men than women have ulcers).

Because these functions are the only ones that are sex-related, the divisions of professions can be explained in terms of temperament: lawyers, managers, MPs and analysts tend to be men, using their thinking function. Women, using their feeling function for social contact, tend to be nurses, social workers and counsellors.

Judging/perceiving

The last pair is that of 'attitudes' to surroundings. Here people are either **judging** (J) or **perceiving** (P). (The words 'judging' and 'perceiving' can be misleading: 'judging' refers rather to concluding; 'perceiving' refers rather to 'becoming aware'.) In this case the question to ask yourself to find out which type you are is this: do you prefer things to be closed and settled, or do you prefer to keep options open and fluid? Do you always know which train you will catch (J), or do you go to the station and take whichever train happens to go (P)? There seems to be no clear distinction in the population for either of these types, and people are about evenly divided between them.

Judging people like things settled, orderly, planned and completed. They plan ahead, make lists and follow them, and get things moving.

Perceiving people, on the other hand, seem to 'play'. They don't like planning, preparing or clearing up. They are flexible, adapt as they go, are tentative and will delay making decisions, hoping always that something better will turn up.

Briggs Myers (1980) describes the 'gifts' which each of these types has, the gifts of judgement being (among others) a system in doing things, order in possessions, sustained effort, acceptance of routine. Some of the gifts of perception are spontaneity, open-mindedness, tolerance, curiosity and adaptability.

It may be difficult for you to decide into which of these two types you fall; with this pair in particular there is a sense of not knowing what is the natural tendency, what you should do, and what you actually do. What you *naturally* do is the right choice.

Awareness of character traits

The conclusion from these simple outlines is that there is a great variety both of people and temperaments. Myers and Briggs have detailed sixteen types. They are called by the letters corresponding to each of the significant words: ESTP, ISTP, ENFJ, ISFP, ENTJ, INTP, and so on.

The significance of this typing is in helping us to recognise a person's character traits. These determine his or her choices, values, and way of living and acting. But a simple outline of any system of categorising the temperaments cannot do justice to all the important elements of psychological typing. In particular it cannot distinguish the significant aspects of personal, social and cultural background. The importance of the exercise is however to see the possibilities: you are the person you are because and in spite of all your personal luggage. Learning or knowing what is in the shadow for you gives you the power to develop your potentialities.

Stephanie

Stephanie was an experienced ward sister who got on well with her colleagues. However, she had difficulties with Sandra, one of the consultants. Stephanie was, according to the Myers–Briggs Type Indicator, an ISFJ (introverted, sensing, feeling, judging). Her knowledge of the typing made her understand that Sandra was ESTP (extraverted, sensing, thinking, perceiving).

I v. E: Stephanie would often see herself as inferior to Sandra, and therefore not speak out when she really wanted to. Once she had not contradicted Sandra on a particular matter, she found it twice as hard to stand up to her the next time. Sandra, on the other hand, did not consider it necessary to ask whether Stephanie had any questions: she assumed that everybody could speak their mind easily.

S: Both were sensing people, practical and observant of patients' conditions. At that level they respected each other's work.

F v. T: Stephanie would consider a patient's whole situation: their illness, their family, the values they had expressed, the meaning they gave to their present predicament, and the relationship she and her staff had with a particular patient. Sandra would see a condition, a set of treatments, and an outcome. She could not understand Stephanie's 'airy fairy' talk. Stephanie found Sandra cold and calculating.

One day Stephanie had phoned Sandra to request that she came and visited a particular patient who was in great pain. Sandra promised to come within the hour. When four hours later she phoned to say she could not come until tomorrow, Stephanie did not insist. She went home and tormented herself about her inability to make Sandra understand her own point of view.

J v. P: The judging function in Stephanie made her value a job well finished, knowing that all was done before she started on something new. Sandra however set no great store by deadlines, and when an unexpected situation turned up she followed that. Sandra could never be pinned down, and this annoyed Stephanie, though she recognised that that particular quality was valued by the patients with whom Sandra would sometimes spend a lot of time, never giving the impression that she had anything else to do.

Because Stephanie knew her typing she was aware of her strengths, particularly her caring attitude with patients and staff. One of the characteristics was an even temper. She knew that some of this was due to her introversion. She found her biggest problem to be a strict judging attitude. This often led her to believe that others ought to be like her: tidy, methodical and always punctual. But she had to learn that not everybody was like that, and once she was able to see — with the help of an empathic friend — that she herself might gain by being less strict with herself, she found that she got on even better with other people, especially Sandra.

She was able to acknowledge Sandra's different characteristics as strengths and learned to work with them rather than let herself be dominated by them. Sandra responded positively to this change by becoming less 'bossy' and more of a colleague.

An awareness of temperament can be a great help. The real help however is knowing what the *shadow*, the undeveloped part, is. Just as towards evening the sun casts longer shadows, so as we grow older our 'shadow' becomes longer, and more apparent to ourselves and others. The challenge is to deal with it.

- If you have decided which type you are, what does that say to you?
- Now think of the person you live/work with most closely.
  – What type is that person according to this simple outline?
  – What are your main differences?
  Look at them, and study the differences, particularly the positive sides.

In my dream I was met by a person whom I knew yet did not recognise. In the symbolic language of dreams this simply means that I met my shadow, that known yet unknown part of me which is also the 'higher self', the soul; that part which completes me and, when listened to, will guide and help me to see where I am, what is happening, and where to go.

Awareness of other people

'No man is an island' is another simple statement which takes a lifetime to unravel and come to grips with.

Volumes have been written on who and what the 'other', the 'neighbour' is. I would like to do no more here than raise the subject as a prelude to much allusion in this book to 'others'.

The objection to self-awareness put by many people is that it leads to introspection and self-centredness. This objection is mainly a fear, and a distorted idea of self-awareness. True awareness leads not to selfishness but to a deeper understanding of people in general, and of how relationships function. A true knowledge of self leads to a true knowledge of others.

One of the benefits of personality indicators is this knowledge of how other people function. To realise that another person has *other* aims and needs, interests, feelings and values than our own can and should release us from our own need to change the world and everything and everyone in it. Instead we can get on with living the life we have more effectively and more contentedly — and *perhaps* help another to live his or her life more effectively too. We cease to be 'directors' of others and instead become 'enablers'. (See the book in this series on *Managing People*.)

Awareness of others will also lead to our being more at ease, knowing and accepting how others see us and how they respond to us and to our presentation of ourselves. In relation to awareness and self-knowledge, the answer to the question 'What's in it for me?' is: a happier and more fulfilled life. How these two words apply to your life depends on you and your interpretation of them. I hope that this book will help you to clarify what they *might* mean for you.

In order to manage yourself well you need to be aware of yourself *and* all that and those who surround you; your body *and* your feelings; your strengths *and* your shadowy needs. You have the choice: to manage yourself or be managed (and used) by them; to be free yourself and to free others, or to be enslaved by yourself and all that surrounds you.

References

1 Briggs Myers, I. 1980. *Gifts Differing*. (Palo Alto, CA: Consulting Psychologists Press Inc., 58, 71, 159.)
2 Gibran, K. 1926. *The Prophet*. (London: Heinemann, 1980 edn, p. 38.)
3 Keirsey, D. and M. Bates, 1984. *Please Understand Me*. (Del Mar, CA: Prometheus Nemesis, pp. 16, 17.)
4 Lefébure, M. 1985. *Human Experience and the Art of Counselling*. (Edinburgh: T. & T. Clark, p. 49.)

Chapter 2   Valuing yourself

'You know what it is until someone asks you to define it', said St. Augustine of time. The same can be said of much else in life. You think you know your values, until someone asks you what they are.

In this chapter and elsewhere in this book I am outlining theories and viewpoints; some are other people's, but all are my own choice. I would like you to see them not as 'laws' but as catalysts or pointers for *your* own choice of values and ideas.

Personal values

- Look at the pictures on pages 11 and 12.
- Decide which one you prefer.
- What does this picture say about yourself?
- Does it evoke memories, depict how you feel, show you what you mean by beauty, invite you to imitate, give you a sense of peace?
- Settle on one reason why you have chosen this picture and revel in your choice. Let the picture speak to you.

From the earlier outline of the temperaments it can be seen that not everyone will find this exercise easy. Thinking people need facts, not imagination, to function. But all of us have **memories**, make **associations**, and have **dreams** about the future. These three elements form the basis for the **esteem** in which we hold ourselves and the **values** we place on concepts and facts.

- What *memory* (e.g. of an illness, or of your home life) has particularly shaped your life?
- What memory has particularly shaped a value that you hold?

- What *association* is now shaping your life? (For example, look again at pages 11 and 12. Does any one photo evoke in you some current concern?)
- What association is shaping a value that you hold?

- What *dream* of the future is particularly shaping your life? (For example, you might wish to be a lecturer in physiology and be taking courses in the subject.)
- What dream of the future is particularly shaping a value for you?

Viktor Frankl (1963) argues that the most important goal in life for a person is the search for **meaning**. He says that 'we can discover this meaning in life in three different ways: (1) by doing a deed, (2) by experiencing a value, (3) by suffering.' Thus we have *creative* values, which we discover through doing or achieving; *experiential* values, which we discover by experiencing something – such as a work of nature or culture – and also by experiencing someone; and *attitudinal* values, which we discover when confronted with something inescapable or unavoidable, such as our own and other people's suffering.

A point which Frankl makes strongly is that we *discover* the meaning of life and in life: we do not create it. Hence the importance of awareness of ourselves, our surroundings and of other people. He illustrates this by saying that 'a cancer which can be cured by surgery must not be shouldered by the patient as though it were his cross. This would be masochism rather than heroism. But if a

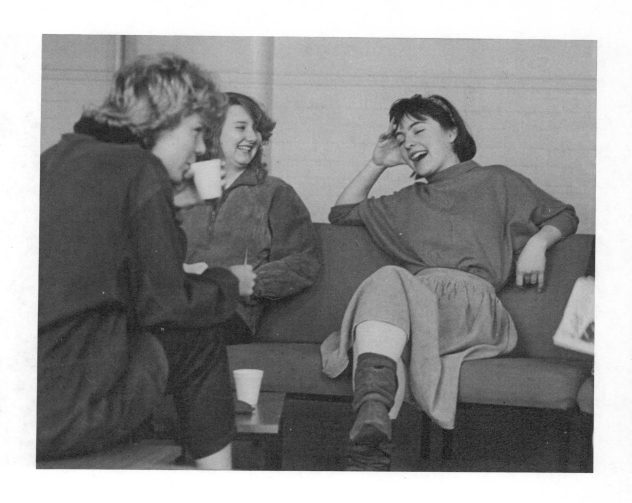

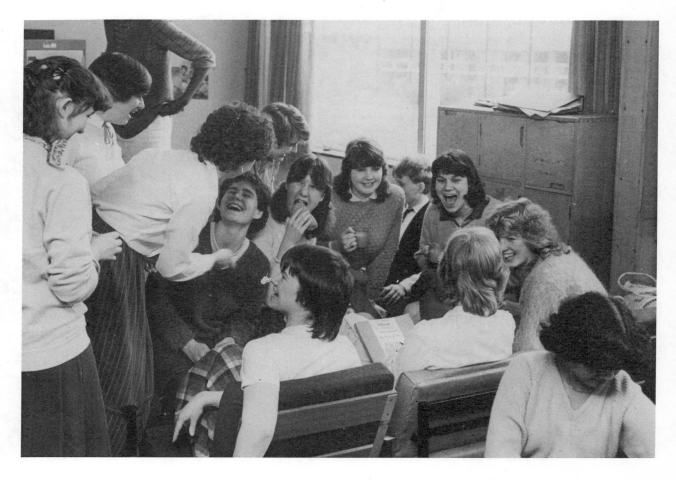

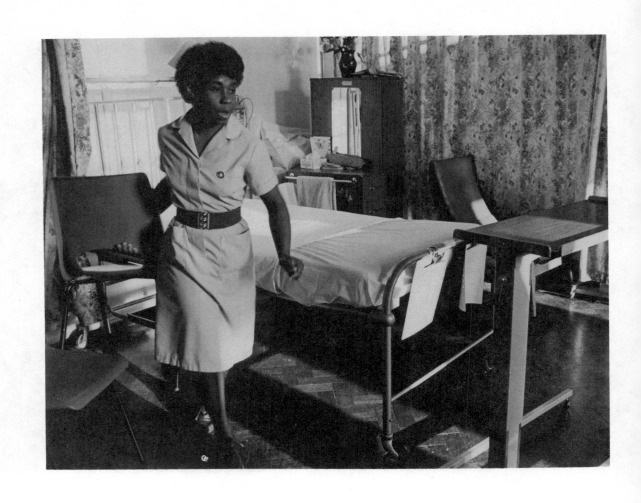

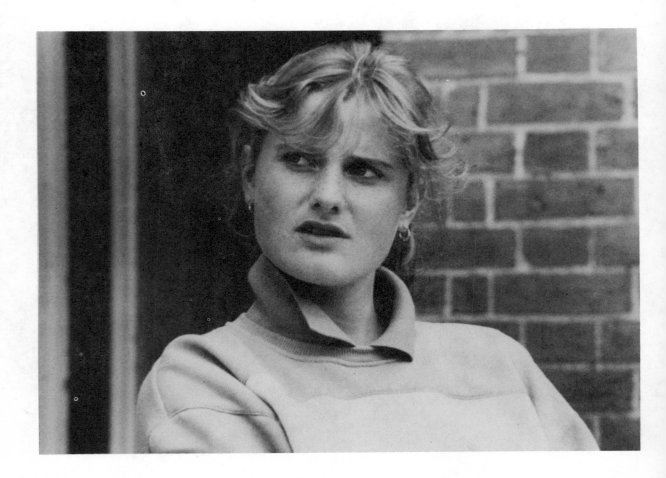

doctor can neither heal the disease nor bring relief to the patient by easing his pain, he should enlist the patient's capacity to fulfil the meaning of his suffering'. This latter applies particularly to nurses also.

Values are changing elements in our lives. They are dynamic, and there is usually an element of motivation involved. But values are built on other factors, such as beliefs and attitudes.

Beliefs are often based on faith rather than facts. We believe that we are going to get home safely tonight; we have no facts to substantiate this.

Attitudes are settled dispositions. They are constant feelings which give order and shape to our lives. We have an attitude of caring, of gratitude, of courtesy. Such an attitude shows what kind of person someone is.

Values then are based on these two pillars. Because we believe that sick people should be cared for whatever their circumstances, we show this in the way we care. This care leads us to conform to certain rules; perhaps at some stage to challenge these rules because circumstances have changed; and because we have changed through the care we gave. Our personal values (memories, associations, dreams) together shape our life: personal, societal and professional values cannot be separated. There may however be conflict when a *personal* value, such as believing that a particular patient should be allowed to die, conflicts with a *professional* value, which demands that all patients have to be resuscitated.

A person who values herself or himself is a person of integrity, that is, someone who does not change 'with every wind of doctrine'. This is certainly not easy in today's world. Part of managing yourself is therefore to have a value-basis that you know and feel comfortable with.

- You might like to ask yourself:
     What is the meaning of your life?
  There may be more than one meaning, or you may not have a ready answer.
- You might like to stay with that question and your answer, as similar questions will come up throughout the book.

The values which you have listed on page 10 may also be applied to Frankl's creative, experiential and attitudinal values. You might like to compare your answers with these expressions.

Values which are right for one person are not necessarily right for another; hence the possibility of conflict. And values emerge and change as we change and the world around us changes.

One nurse's values	When I trained as a nurse I had egg and bacon for breakfast every day. When I had to pay for it, I had it less often. When cholesterol became an issue, I gave it up. With time I became a vegetarian, not liking to eat anything which has to be killed for food. But *my* value does not mean that *everybody* has to have it too.
	On the other hand it is now clear that the hole in the ozone layer is getting bigger due to CFCs. By using certain hairsprays I contribute directly to the destruction of life on this planet. The value of life – and beauty – is compromised, and by every means possible I should see that no harmful sprays are used by me *or* by anyone else.

Smith (1977) lists eight questions which may help in clarifying how values come about:

(1) Have I freely chosen this value?
(2) From among what alternatives?
(3) What are the consequences of choosing this value?
(4) How recently have I acted on this value?
(5) In what way has this value become a regular pattern in my life?
(6) When did I most recently publicly affirm this value?
(7) How do I prize or celebrate this value in my life?
(8) How does this value help me to grow as a person?

The essence of these questions is that we have to *choose*, *prize* and *act* on values. We have to be aware of what is given, find the meaning of it, and then do something about it.

What is here?
What is happening? } *Choosing*

What is the meaning of it?
What is your purpose? } *Prizing*

What are you doing about it? *Acting*

Look at the following sentences and complete them, aware, as far as possible, of how you came to hold such a value, what its implications are, and how you would defend it if asked.

- One day I hope to ...
- I enjoy ...
- My work is ...
- People who are well-dressed are ...
- My favourite place is ...
- Elderly people should ...
- The person who influences me most taught me to ...
- If I were ill I would ...
- Artistic beauty is ...
- If I had a million I would ...
- My parents are ...
- Sick people are ...
- I would like to be remembered for ...
- Nuclear weapons should ...
- The people I work with are ...
- Developing and discovering means ...
- My greatest possession is ...
- I am lucky to have ...
- Freedom of speech is ...
- What I would most like to change is ...

You might like to see whether you would have answered these questions differently five years ago, and what has changed for you in the meantime. You might also keep in mind that meaning is not created, but discovered.

Professional values

Under this heading I would like to highlight certain areas of nursing values that I find significant. Look at them critically, and check your own values against them.

Roach (1984) says that 'caring is the locus of all attributes used to describe nursing'. **Caring** is thus not only the main *value* of nursing, but its *essence*. But she sees caring not only as a nursing act; she says that 'to care is human; to be human is to care'. She details her theory by establishing the 'Five Cs' of caring:

- compassion
- competence
- confidence
- conscience
- commitment

Compassion: A way of living born out of an awareness of one's relationship to all living creatures; engendering a response of participation in the experience of another; a sensitivity to the pain and brokenness of the other; a quality of presence which allows one to share with and make room for the other.

Competence: The state of having the knowledge, judgement, skills, energy, experience and motivation required to respond adequately to the demands of one's professional responsibilities.

Confidence: The quality which fosters trusting relationships.

Conscience: A state of moral awareness; a compass directing one's behaviour according to the moral fitness of things.

Commitment: A complex affective response characterised by a convergence between one's desires and one's obligations, and by a deliberate choice to act in accordance with them.

Campbell (1984) adds another dimension to nursing which, co-incidentally, also begins with C: he describes nursing as **companionship**:

The good companion is someone who shares freely but does not impose, allowing others to make their *own* journey. .... Companionship is bodily presence, but not specifically sexual.

14

... The good companion looks ahead and encourages ... The commitment of companionship is a *limited* one ... parting is an essential element in companionship.

If nursing can be summed up as 'caring', and caring is the human mode of being, then nurses should above all 'be', and be human. 'An individual cares, not because he or she is a nurse, but because he or she is a human being' (Roach, 1984).

- How do you respond to these statements?
- Do they represent the values you have of nursing, of yourself as a nurse and as a person?
- What would you change, or add? Make a note of it.

In order to translate these theories into practice, I would like to examine briefly just four areas of nursing which are particularly relevant today.

Professionalism

Nursing is not a profession in the strict sense (such as law, medicine and the Church), but nurses behave in a professional way: they adhere to some common rules and they put their knowledge and skills at the service of others.

Nursing has had a Code of Ethics since 1953. The *Code of Professional Conduct for the Nurse, Midwife and Health Visitor* issued by the United Kingdom Central Council (UKCC) in 1984 has been much discussed and used. A **code**, according to May (1975), 'shapes human behaviour in a fashion somewhat similar to habits and rules'. The Code 'shapes', but it does not 'protect'. Each nurse has to use her own ability to interpret the Code, and in the light of this use her personal and professional responsibility.

According to Pyne (1987), the Code does this in that:

- it gives advice to all those on the registers on the standards of professional conduct;
- it portrays the kind of practitioner the UKCC believes is needed;
- it is the backcloth against which allegations of misconduct are judged;
- it is a weapon for the practitioners with which to fight for improved standards and eliminate risks in the interest of patients;
- it provides an extended definition of accountability;
- it is a statement to the profession of the primacy of the patient's interests.

The values listed above are the UKCC's values.

- Do you agree with them?
- Are you the kind of nurse the UKCC wants?
- When and how do you use the Code?
- Has it shaped your professional values?

May (1975) develops another dimension of professionalism: the idea of **covenant**. According to him, a covenant is 'an original experience of gift between ... partners'. Code and covenant are similar materially, but they differ in spirit. Contracts and codes define relationships, but covenants 'have a gratuitous growing edge to them that nourishes rather than limits relationships'. 'Contracts are external; covenants are internal to the parties involved'. In contracts there is a tit-for-tat; in covenants one *gives*. This is what Roach (1984) is pointing to when she says that to care is human. To be human one has to be creative; giving – responding – is creative.

In the light of these theories you might like to formulate your own list of professional values.

As an example:
- When I am caring, I ...
- As a nurse, I ...
- As myself, I ...

Professional autonomy

If nursing is not a profession, should nurses try so hard to make their mark, research independently, make nursing diagnoses, and to extend and expand their role?

According to the Myers–Briggs Type Indicators, nurses tend to be of the sensing–feeling (SF) type. These people are concerned with order, tradition, harmony, personal values and devotion.

The people who are intuitive, forward-looking and ingenious, who shape the future with their imagination, and the people who think logically and see value in policies, standards and analysis (NT), make up only 7 per cent of the nursing population (Briggs Myers, 1980). This may explain why nursing has such difficulty in establishing itself autonomously.

Autonomy, says Mayeroff (1972), 'is the opposite of both arbitrary behaviour (doing simply as I please) and behaviour controlled by what is basically foreign to me'. Autonomy has much to do with power, and it is in the use of power that true caring is shown. Since autonomy has significantly to do with living the meaning of life, this power is seen in the way we use it to enhance ourselves and those for whom we care.

Mayeroff goes on to say that, 'in order to live "my own life" I must make it my own through caring and taking responsibility for it, just as I must act on an ideal and help to actualize it if I am to make it my own. I am not autonomous to begin with; autonomy is an achievement like maturity or the growth of a significant friendship'. What is said here of the individual is applicable to nursing as a whole: autonomy is not something given; it is achieved in the way in which nurses care. When they do this not as powerful experts, but as companions, then society itself will confer autonomy on nursing just as now it still maintains the image of handmaids and angels.

Advocacy

Curtin (1979) bases a philosophy of nursing on the concept of **advocacy**. She says that an advocate is first and foremost a person who can and does enter into a relationship with another person. Caring relationships are based on human rights, and these in turn derive from human needs. The human rights of life and liberty, and the pursuit of justice, happiness, truth, knowledge, beauty, harmony and so on are needs. Too often, however, needs are confused with wants.

Advocacy implies interest and partnership. An advocate can only act in that role if she or he respects another person and her or his values, means and status. A true advocate does not *represent* a person, but with every means possible helps that person to be not dependent but informed and 'self-advocating'.

The role of advocate is a delicate one. Walsh (1985) believes that there is a deep conflict for the advocate, as to where her or his **loyalties** lie. Is a nurse first of all loyal to the patient (for whom she or he cares), to the doctor (who prescribes the treatment), to the hospital (which employs her or him) or to the profession (who controls her or his registration)?

A psychiatric patient has complained to the nursing staff that her drugs make her feel drowsy and generally unwell. The charge nurse maintains that the patient's views should be taken seriously and medication stopped. The medical staff disagree and continue to prescribe, arguing that her condition will deteriorate if medication is discontinued. The charge nurse takes a stand on the patient's behalf and refuses to administer the drugs.

(Melia, 1987)

- What is your opinion?
- Should the charge nurse have acted as he did?
- Should the medical staff have been more willing to listen?
- What do you think you would have done in this case?
- Have you had some similar experience?
- What did you mainly gain/learn/suffer from such an experience?

Advocacy is not a new concept or slogan. It is one of the basic values of nursing. But the conflicts that it may bring are not easy to resolve. The issues of personal responsibility and awareness of values and meaning are sharply focused here. New concepts, such as self-advocacy (primarily used by minority or under-privileged groups to get a voice) and citizen-advocacy (ordinary people being involved with vulnerable individuals) may also need to be studied and learnt.

- Where in your work is advocacy used, or questioned, or abused?
- How much priority do you give to advocacy?
- Do you see nursing values growing or eroding generally?
- What are you doing to maintain and foster any particular values?

Accountability

Most often **accountability** is linked with quality control and quality assurance. In times of financial stringency everyone is expected to comply with the rules. The one who is given responsibility is made accountable for this.

This is easy enough when it is a question of so many dressing packs issued and so many dressings done. But it is much more difficult to measure the quality of a relationship between patients and nurses, and what goes on in that relationship while a dressing is being performed. Those in charge of the purse-strings have difficulty in measuring the truths told and gifts given in a covenant. May (1975) states that 'covenant fidelity to the patient remains unrealized if it does not include proficiency'. He goes on to say that 'covenant ethics must include rather than exclude the interests of the codes'. Accountability that can be measured in terms of codes and contracts is therefore included in the notion of the covenant. This corresponds with Binnie's (1984) statement that 'accountability may be described as being personally responsible for the outcome of one's own professional actions'.

This brings us back then to self-awareness, to knowledge and autonomy, to one's own values of the meaning of nursing, and to our own understanding and goal of life, of care, of suffering, and where our personal responsibility lies. Without all these aspects, accountability would simply be seen in terms of pounds and pence.

- What value do you place on accountability?
- Where in your caring are you particularly accountable?
- How does this manifest itself?
- Are you satisfied with this?
- If not, what might you or should you do to change it?

There are many other professional issues that are value-laden. Confidentiality, informed consent, private health care and complementary medicine are only some aspects that would need much attention. In your own area of work there will be other issues with their own values.

The dream I recounted at the beginning has some relationship to personal and professional values:

- I responded as a professional to a call of urgency: as professionals, this is our first duty.
- The more I helped, the more people were found: good care will allow more good care to be applied.
- After a while I became aware that lots of people were rushing about but not 'doing' anything: people who have no clear aims or meaning or values tend to be 'rushing about', blown by the wind in this direction and that, not getting anywhere.
- The person who helped me was none other than my 'inner' self, my psyche or soul, which was teaching me not to rush about, but to stop, stay and look at what was happening. Only in this way could I see the meaning of my work as a nurse, prize it, cherish it, get it into a perspective, and act on it by returning to it. Once I could do that I was convinced again of the value of my training, my skills, and my humanity.

You may by now be having your own dream: stay with it and listen to what it says to you; it may help you to define your skills, ideas and values, and to recognise how to manage yourself effectively.

References

1 Binnie, A. (ed.) 1984. *A Systematic Approach to Nursing Care*. (Milton Keynes: Open University Press.)
2 Briggs Myers, I. 1980. *Gifts Differing*. (Palo Alto, CA: Consulting Psychologists Press Inc., pp. 58, 71, 159.)
3 Campbell, A. V. 1984. *Moderated Love*. (London: SPCK, pp. 49–50.)
4 Curtin, L. L. 1979. 'The nurse as advocate: a philosophical foundation for nursing.' *Advances in Nursing Science* **1**(3), pp. 1–10.
5 Frankl, V. 1963. *Man's Search for Meaning*. (London: Hodder & Stoughton, pp. 113, 115.)
6 May, W. F. 1975. 'Code, covenant, contract, or philanthropy'. *Hastings Center Report* **5**, pp. 29–38.
7 Mayeroff, M. 1972. *On Caring*. (New York: Harper & Row, p. 80.)
8 Melia, K. 1987. 'Whose side are you on?' *Nursing Times* **83**(29), pp. 46–8.
9 Pyne, R. 1987. 'A professional duty to shout.' *Nursing Times* **83**(42), pp. 30–1.
10 Roach, M. S. 1984. *Caring: the Human Mode of Being, Implications for Nursing*. Perspectives in Caring Monograph 1. (Toronto: University of Toronto.)
11 Smith, M. 1977. *A Practical Guide to Value Clarification*. (La Jolla, CA: University Associates, p. 69.)
12 UKCC 1984. *Code of Professional Conduct for the Nurse, Midwife and Health Visitor* (2nd edn.). (London: United Kingdom Central Council.)
13 Walsh, P. 1985. 'Speaking up for the patient'. *Nursing Times* **81**(18), pp. 24–6.

Chapter 3   Motivating yourself

What determines the ethical value of our actions is never the materiality of the external act but strictly the 'heart', the basic dispositions and value-responses which can be the source of ethical good as well as evil.

(Häring, 1978)

Your values will eventually manifest themselves — your **motives** may not. They remain your private property. This is why they are so elusive, yet so crucial: your management of yourself depends on them.

A man was walking along a river when he saw a person coming towards him in the river, about to drown. The man pulled the person out and resuscitated him. As he walked on, another victim, about to drown, was in the river, and he helped this one out too. And so on with a third and fourth. After this he got up, to the astonishment of the onlookers, who chided him for not rescuing all the victims who were coming downstream. As he walked away, the man said, 'I am going upstream to see who or what throws the people in.'

(Egan and Cowan, 1979)

Motivation

What makes you get up in the morning and not sleep on? Is it the call of duty, or hunger, or a meeting you are looking forward to? The alarm clock waking you up is the external stimulus; the internal stimulus is some drive, some hope, some call, some need.

Motivation has been described as 'the tendency of the organism to reduce its needs or to return to its state of equilibrium' (Stones, 1966). This is too mechanistic a view. We do not eat only in order to quench hunger. We eat also for desire, for circumstances and for feelings.

O'Connor (1968) lists some of the general reasons for motivation:

- genuine interest
- a wish to perform the task well
- conforming to a standard
- looking for approval from superiors
- looking for recognition from colleagues
- in order to please
- in order not to disappoint
- a better salary if success is achieved

Simonton *et al.* (1978) found that cancer patients who in the degree of their well-being had beaten every statistic often made statements like, ' "I can't die until my son graduates from college", or "They need me too much at work", or "I won't die until I've solved the problem with my daughter". The common thread running through these replies was the belief that they exerted some influence over the course of their disease.'

Motivation consists of both external and internal factors. An external weighing-up of a situation, making an **estimate**, leads to an internal situation of **esteem**. That in turn leads to the response that characterises a person.

The stimulus for the man who resuscitated people was presumably that he was fed up with resuscitating people. That led him to question what he was doing. His esteem for himself made him get up and do something positive. Knowing how slowly and laboriously institutions move, it may then have taken him a long time to achieve his goal: that no more people were thrown in!

From the estimate to the esteem, from the external stimulus to the motivation or 'heart', may be a long road. The self-respect that is generated is based in that feeling of being of value, and out of that comes the response to the stimulus.

- What are motivators for you? (Examples include a certificate, a gift, the knowledge of having done right.)
- When were you last motivated to make a significant break or change? What was the stimulus? Did it see you through the change?

Lucy

Lucy was a shy 16-year-old who was underweight and often sick. A well-meaning neighbour gave her a leaflet about pilgrimages to Lourdes, and Lucy's parents – in an effort to try everything – paid for her to go. There she mingled with sick people of all ages, some very handicapped. They all looked well, however. Lucy became more companionable, decided to train as a nurse, and years later still used her memory of the looks on the pilgrims' faces to give herself and her patients courage.

- What was your reason or motive for going into nursing?
- What keeps you there now? (You might like to make a note of it.)
- What or which personal or professional value do you recognise as motivating you most in your work as a nurse?
  - money/security;
  - the need to be needed;
  - an impossibility of changing jobs;
  - exerting control;
  - influencing others;
  - giving of yourself to others;
  - being looked up to;
  - altruism;
  - following the example of a charismatic person.
- Can you identify a particular standard that you want to or have to maintain?
  - a standard of care;
  - self-respect;
  - respect for others;
  - control;
  - justice;
  - autonomy;
  - honesty.
- Is this in yourself or in others?
- Is it more important that it is
  - in yourself?
  - in others?
- How much are you in charge of yourself and your work? How much are other people in charge (making policies, giving directives)?

The man in the story changed from responding to what was simply there, to responding to a deeper insight. That must have changed the whole direction of his life. Once he had gone upstream he had some control over what he was doing – before then the situation controlled him.

You may have known your values and acted on them. If and when you are confronted with a choice at some stage, you may simply not recognise your value, or know your 'mind'. Your motives may be unclear. Your meaning, your 'leitmotiv', is questioned. This may be more of a challenge than a disaster. Like the rescuer, you may suddenly discover what lies potentially within you.

Mistakes and failures

Mistakes may be painful for all concerned. With every good intention we still make mistakes, and skilled as we are at certain tasks, we still fail. Mistakes and failures then become positive or negative motivators. We either change, or we drift into apathy.

D. H. Lawrence is supposed to have said this: 'If only one could have two lives: the first in which to make one's mistakes, which seem as if they have to be made; and the second in which to profit by them.' Often we learn more from our mistakes than in any other way. The learning comes when it is interiorised, acknowledged and owned.

The basis of mistakes and failures

The temperament is an important element in the understanding of mistakes and failures.

Sensing people put much emphasis on history, past events and facts. They tend to dwell on their past, and can recount and relive events leading up to an accident or disaster over and over again. Their intuitive personality is in the shadow, and therefore they do not trust the future and will rather stay with 'the devil they know'.

Intuitive people on the other hand have a poor memory for history, and they will get up and go forward. Consequently they may be inclined not to learn from mistakes because they pay little attention to the past.

Our personalities are shaped by our association with other people and with the environment in which we live and work. We are influenced and we let ourselves be influenced. We know this and realise it, but often do not acknowledge it.

When we make **mistakes** we make them out of the shadow, out of that part of the personality which is not well developed or known, or controlled. This is why we get so furious when we make a mistake: we recognise that the mistake shows up the infantile, weak and incompetent part of ourselves.

Failure is different. A mistake has to be admitted; failure has to be lived with. Neither mistakes nor failure are wrong, or wrong-doing. But a deliberately wrong action cannot be called a mistake: it is more than that.

A failure on the whole is not based on a particular mistake, but rather on a series of events that have negatively influenced a person. The people in the story who were about to drown could be described as failures: failures of their own values and hopes, and failures of the system in which they found themselves. Yet people in themselves are not failures: that would be to condemn them. But events around them have influenced their behaviour and particularly their will — their motivation — and rather than struggle forward, they have taken the easy way and drifted down with the tide.

Judging a failure as such — in ourselves and others — is subjective. The values we place on making judgements, on failures and on successes, will colour any outcome.

We have to live with past failures. But we do not have to live and *perpetuate* a failure. Failures need to be seen in perspective, as a natural part of human living and growing. Like mistakes, they can be incentives to change and adapt and learn. Because they have to do with the shadowy, undeveloped part of ourselves, failures give us a possibility either of developing that side of ourselves, or of strengthening further the strong part of the personality. Either possibility can be right at the right time.

Renewed motivation

Mistakes and failures are painful. They lead to dark times in life when we feel dejected, lonely and helpless. They lead to loss of confidence and make us question any motives we had.

Yet such times seem essential also. When values become uncertain, when skills are doubted, and when any self-esteem is absent, that is the moment when we are faced with ourselves. The question 'What is the meaning of it?' is then the only relevant question. As light has meaning only in darkness, so the real meaning of life is usually discovered only in a crisis. Once the meaning of something is discovered, the motivation for change, for direction, or for defying any predictions is there. But change does not happen of its own. We have to take a personal responsibility for it.

The motivation in my dream for getting back to work is not obvious. But the element of crisis and of failure is there, out of which grew the motivation and the change. In the act of sitting down and feeling the failure and the tears, I came to see that I am not suited to work in a disaster. The realisation of that was painful. It gave me the insight that I am more suited to the slower work with patients in a ward (not casualties). Once that had sunk in – once I had personally taken the responsibility for this insight – I was ready to have a wash and put on a new uniform: the 'uniform' of the new mind, the new insight, became the motivation which led me back to work rather than stay sitting in the rubble.

References

1 Egan, G. and R. M. Cowan 1979. *People and Systems*. (Belmont, CA: Brooks/Cole, p. 140.)
2 Häring, B. 1978. *Free and Faithful in Christ*, Vol. I. (Middlegreen: St. Paul Publications, p. 94.)
3 O'Connor, K. 1968. *Learning: an introduction*. (London: Macmillan, p. 31.)
4 Simonton, O. C., S. Mathews–Simonton and J. L. Creighton, 1978. *Getting Well Again*. (New York: Bantam Books, p. 5.)
5 Stones, E. 1966. *An Introduction to Educational Psychology*. (London: Methuen, p. 97.)

22

Chapter 4   Asserting yourself

An assertive person is one who gets his or her needs and wants met without stepping on the rights of others.

(Egan, 1977)

Assertiveness has come to the fore with the feminist movement, and is sometimes seen to be something peculiar to women. In practice, however, this is not true. Many men do not know how to use assertiveness, being more familiar with a commanding and aggressive type of behaviour.

Being assertive is nothing more and nothing less than being a good communicator. It is using oneself and the other person in such a way that both are enhanced and valued. When this happens good management of human resources has taken place.

Aggression or assertion?

Assertiveness has to do with expressing feelings, needs, wants and rights.

Egan (1977) says that there are three different ways in which people express their emotions:

(1) Non-assertively — you just take it.
(2) Aggressively — you teach him a lesson.
(3) Assertively — you let him know how you feel without punishing him.

Bond (1986) lists four approaches to expressing yourself:

(1) assertive;
(2) aggressive;
(3) manipulative;
(4) submissive.

Each of these approaches is legitimate in its right setting. A person doesn't always need to get her or his way, have the last word, or make others submit. Courtesy and manners, sometimes a dose of humility (not humiliation), and letting things be as they are, are also called for. But when none of these approaches is constructive, then assertiveness usually is.

The **submissive** way of being is one of appeasing. 'Would you mind —? . . . I mean, could you possibly —? . . . If I asked you nicely —? . . . Forgive me . . . .' This is flattering the other, making her or him big and yourself small. We imagine that a 'big bully' will respond to us better if we enhance this bigness.

Being **passive** is taking things lying down, giving in. Even though we feel strong emotions, we say nothing. Later, though, we may burst into tears and in this way ensure that we are noticed and can tell our hard-luck story, blaming everyone and everything.

The **indirect** or **manipulative** approach can be hurtful but doesn't wound. It is an underhand, backlashing way, revealing an insecure personality. Double messages may be given: too friendly, too secure, too concerned. But when it is all over, what remains is guilt — in the other person, of course. People never quite know how to approach such a person, because he or she never 'comes clean' in any situation.

The **aggressive** person bloats herself or himself up to twice the size, hands on hips. The body language alone would say everything, but that is not enough: shouting, long tirades and verbal abuse are also the stock-in-trade to get what is wanted. Those around are careful (submissive) in case they provoke such a person even further. This alienates everybody, making each think that they are right and everybody else is wrong.

The **assertive** way of being and responding to emotions is everything else! You know what is going on, you remain cool, people do what you ask because you respect them — and they respect you. You don't *blame* others for what happens to you. You know what you need and want. If you are refused something, you are not demolished by it. You can respond to criticism because you can judge how valid it is.

In order to clarify any unproductive types of behaviour it is useful to look at feelings, body language, needs, rights and wants in turn. In this way you may see where you may want or need to make adjustments in your own style of communication.

Aspects of behaviour

Feelings

Feelings are powerful – and delicate – things which can either make or mar a relationship. Feelings are experienced in the body but expressed in words – or not, as the case may be.

Letting feelings rule you altogether means that either you are in the clouds or in the dumps or you are verbally abusive. Neither approach by itself is ideal: as usual a middle way would be preferable.

One simple method of finding this middle way is to learn how to distinguish feelings, how to express them, and what other words we might find for similar feelings. Table 4.1 may help you with this. Please add to the lists your own appropriate words.

Table 4.1 Different types of feelings and different strengths of expression of feelings

	Happy	*Sad*	*Angry*	*Confused*
Strong	excited elated	hopeless depressed	furious seething	bewildered troubled
Moderate	cheerful merry	upset distressed	annoyed mad	disorganised mixed-up
Weak	glad pleased	sorry bad	uptight irritated	bothered undecided

(Tschudin, 1989)

When you can *name* a thing – a feeling – then you have some control over it. This does not mean suppressing it: feelings of deep sorrow are best expressed through tears; feelings of deep joy through laughter.

Feelings are simply there. They cannot be explained, and they cannot be explained away. A typical mistake is to counter them with reason.

Anne

Anne, a senior staff nurse (and a feeling-type person) saw the need for some small changes in the way patients were admitted to the ward. She felt that in this way everybody, patients, relatives and staff, would benefit. Ron, the charge nurse (a thinking-type person) listened to her, but did not believe that the changes would really change anything. Anne tried again, but as Ron shook his head, she sniped, 'If only you would be a bit more feeling!' This annoyed him, and he walked off with, 'If only *you* would learn to be logical!'

Once you are aware of your feelings you can choose what to do with them: express them or control them. That choice is the most important element. Assertiveness in particular, and communication skills in general, are based on the ability to make that choice.

The further choice is between *sharing* your emotions and *releasing* them.

Your colleague says to you: 'You've filled that form in wrong again. Can't you ever get anything right?'

Your choice in answering is between:
(1) 'I feel hurt and put down. I spent a lot of time filling in this form.'
(2) 'Don't you shout at me! You don't know what you do to people with these remarks of yours.'

The release of emotion can happen in a controlled or uncontrolled way. You know what you are doing and saying, or you are flying off the handle. Anger in particular is often expressed in an uncontrolled way, but then lasts only a short while before it is burnt up. Swallowed, however, it may go on for many years, poisoning the person and her or his environment.

● Which is your most usual way of dealing with strong emotion?
● Are you content with this, or would you like to change?
● Make a note of the change you might like to make, and in the light of this chapter (and the book *Managing Change* in this series) see how you might bring this change about.

Body language

Assertiveness is about communication. **Body language** is the most basic and most obvious way we have of communicating.

Be aware right now of how you are sitting or standing. What is this posture saying to you and about you?

Our gestures often speak louder about us and for us than do our words. Our bodies reveal our thoughts, our attitudes and our desires. We can let them do this consciously, but in moments of crisis they do it without our knowing. Here are some common expressions of feelings:
● In embarrassment people may cover their mouths.
● In anger they may lean forward.
● In sadness they may turn sideways.
● When encroached on they may move back.
● When thinking hard they may put their tongues out a little.
● When experiencing envy they may become 'green'.
● When being submissive they may bend at the knee.
● When talking deeply they may look away.

Feelings may be swallowed or 'hidden', but the body can reveal them more than words can. People who are anxious or embarrassed often giggle. People put on an air of relaxation when they are seething with rage. To give such confused or mixed messages can be deliberate or unconscious.

Patients are people under stress. They may therefore not behave 'as themselves'. As the person caring for them, you don't know what a patient was before he or she became ill; you have only the present to go by. How good are you at interpreting their put-on signals, their masks or their defences?

As a nurse you are a privileged person: few family members can or would touch a person all over the body. You have the patient's unspoken (usually) agreement to invade her or his space. Some people welcome this, others resent it. The sexual connotations are legion, and nurses are not depicted as 'sex-objects' for nothing.

When you are caring for a patient, are you aware of the signals you are giving with your face when there is odour, disfigurement, like, dislike? Patients enjoy nothing so much as 'nurse-watching'.

Needs

Needs are another knowledge-base for effective assertion. Maslow (1970) established five 'needs', which he expressed in the form of a pyramid:

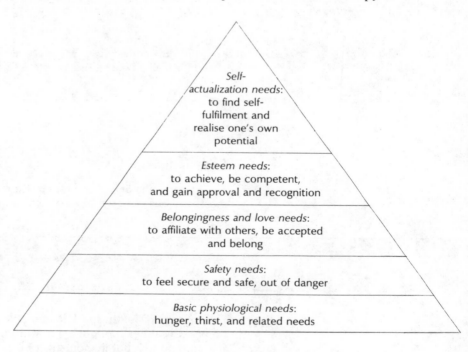

These needs are basic to life, though the higher ones can only be fulfilled if the lower ones are met. People who have to spend their lives meeting the lower needs have no energy left for either esteem or self-actualisation needs.

Our needs constantly change.

Look at the pyramid, and be aware of yourself. What is your need at this moment?
- to make a cup of coffee?
- to get the electrician to fix the faulty plug?
- to phone a friend and tell her or him what sort of a day you had?
- to finish reading this book?
- to compose the poem which has been growing in you for the last few days?

When you *know* your actual needs you are able to cater for them. If you don't cater for them, they get out of proportion.

Needs are closely related to motivation. Getting your needs fulfilled is an incentive: needs motivate you. In the manner in which you treat your needs lies the clue to what 'makes you tick'.

Rights

Rights, or fair claims, arise straight out of needs and are another of those bases for assertiveness. Rights are things we are entitled to. According to the Declaration of Independence of the United States of America, we have the 'inalienable' right to 'life, liberty and the pursuit of happiness'. Seeing this in the light of assertiveness gives you kudos and certainty. Dickson (1982) lists eleven rights that a person has with regard to assertiveness. These are:

the right to
- state my own needs and set my own priorities as a person independent of any roles that I may assume in my life;
- to be treated with respect as an intelligent, capable and equal human being;
- to express my feelings;
- to express my opinions and values;
- to say 'yes' or 'no' for myself;
- to make mistakes;
- to change my mind;
- to say I don't understand;
- to ask for what I want;
- to decline responsibility for other people's problems;
- to deal with others without being dependent on them for approval.

Perls, the founder of Gestalt therapy, wrote this 'prayer' (1973).

I am I,
And you are you.
I'm not in this world to
live up to your expectations.
And you're not in this world
to live up to mine.
I is I.
And you is you.

Knowing and recognising your rights literally means knowing and recognising **boundaries**. In that way you don't step on the rights of other people; and they don't step on yours: you are preventing them from stepping on your boundaries. Your responsibility is for yourself and *your* problems, not for others' problems.

You might like to repeat the Gestalt prayer and memorise it. It might come in useful in times of stress, conflict, or even having to make a decision whether to interiorise a feeling or to make it explicit.

Wants

Wants are strong feelings and are often confused with needs or rights. A person in an out-patients' department who has been waiting for a long time may assert the right to be seen 'now', but that is neither a right nor a need, but a want or desire.

We hear much said these days about rights, and most of these 'rights' are really egoistic wants. We are used to the idea that when we turn a switch we will get light: in the same way we think our needs should be satisfied. When considering assertive behaviour we need to be sure that we know the difference between needs and wants.

As a nurse you may *want* many things which could improve your lot and that of the patients. You may have to weigh these against the actual needs and possibilities. Otherwise your assertiveness will only be criticised and ridiculed. To know clearly the difference between your desires and your needs may indeed be your most potent form of assertiveness.

Are you assertive?

Egan (1986) has outlined three 'Think Steps' for performing certain behaviours. Adapted to assertiveness, their essence is as follows:

At the 'Before' Think Step, stop and ask yourself:
- Do I know what I need?
- Do I know what I am going to say about myself?
- Am I open (not pre-judging a person or a situation)?
- Am I feeling sure of myself (not rejected)?

At the 'During' Think Step, stop and ask yourself:
- Am I being myself (or what I think 'they' expect me to be)?
- Am I listening, trying to understand the other's point of view?
- Am I ready to accept some negative signs without letting them get me down, or blaming someone?
- I have a choice of how to deal with my feelings — am I ready to choose the better way?

At the 'After' Think Step, stop and ask yourself:
- Am I letting myself get depressed that everything did not go perfectly?
- Is there anything I would like to add or say now?
- Is there anything I would like to question the other person about?

Advice on how to remain cool abounds:

- counting to ten;
- taking a few deep breaths;
- remembering your home telephone number;
- saying a prayer;
- thinking of the other person as an island — you sail right round it and only then land on it.

Such tactics give you space to become aware of yourself. They also give you the space to ask yourself:

- what is happening?
- what is the meaning of it?
- what am I going to do about it (see Chapter 2)?

The areas in which being assertive is — or can be — difficult have been well outlined by Bond (1986), and are hinted at in the Think Steps. They are mainly to do with:

- making a request;
- saying no;
- making a point;
- setting limits;
- giving feedback;
- responding to feedback.

Below are assertive statements relating to each of the above topics. Make your own assertive remark for each, taking a situation that is familiar to you.

- *Making a request*: 'I need to know where I stand on this. Could you phone me before 5 p.m. with your answer, please?'

- *Saying no*: 'No thank you, I don't want to buy any more tickets now.'

- *Making a point*: 'I find your description fascinating. I think that you have, however, overlooked one area which concerns me particularly.'

- *Setting limits*: 'Yes, this *is* my free weekend, but I want it for myself this time.'

- *Giving feedback*: 'You look great in that dress. You know how to enhance your figure with your choices.'

- *Responding to feedback*: 'You spotted that mistake rightly, but I don't agree with you that I make it all the time.'

The following is a set of aggressive, manipulative and (generally) non-assertive statements. Try making the same point in an assertive way.

- 'You make me so angry; no wonder I shout at you.'
- 'We have a no-smoking policy around here; can't you see the signs?'
- 'Mind your own business. Who told you to teach me my own job?'
- 'You never seem to learn how to listen.'

Assertiveness is not really difficult — in fact it is surprisingly easy. When you have been assertive a few times you come to value yourself much more, feel in charge and respect yourself, and that makes you respect others. Your whole network of relationships changes to one of confidence. This gives **courage** and invites **trust** and **honesty**. Once you feel less trapped in a role, doing things this way because you have always done them this way, then you also release others from *their* traps. Assertiveness is putting into practice what you believe and value about yourself and others.

Assertiveness in nurses is often equated with patient advocacy (see Chapter 2). To speak up for the patient is indeed good, and too often in the past nurses have *not* spoken up for various reasons, fear being the most cogent. But a nurse can only do this if she or he has been given permission by the patient. If the nurse takes on this task without permission, this is stepping on the patient's rights. Speaking up for patients means first of all speaking *with* them, hearing their story, values, and motives.

It was clear in my dream that I hadn't asserted myself. I went along to the emergency not knowing and not respecting my feelings, needs, rights or wants. I went because it was expected of me. The downfall therefore seems inevitable: I didn't assert myself, and instead stressed myself.

Moral: Not to be stressed, be assertive.

References

1 Bond, M. 1986. *Stress and Self-Awareness: a guide for nurses*. (London: Heinemann, pp. 100, 104, 173, 213.
2 Dickson, A. 1982. *A Woman in Your Own Right*. (London: Quartet Books, p. 29.)
3 Egan, G. 1977. *You & Me*. (Monterey, CA: Brooks/Cole, pp. 78, 267.)
4 Egan, G. 1986. *The Skilled Helper* (3rd edn). (Monterey, CA: Brooks/Cole, p. 341.)
5 Maslow, A. 1970. *Motivation and Personality* (2nd edn). (New York: Harper & Row.)
6 Perls, F. 1973. *The Gestalt Approach and Eye Witness to Therapy*. (New York: Bantam Books, p. 141.)
7 Tschudin, V. 1989. *Beginning with Empathy*. (Edinburgh: Churchill Livingstone.)

Chapter 5

Stressing yourself

Stress and stressors

If people say they are stressed or exhibit stress symptoms, they should be believed. What *feels* real has a basis in reality.

(McNeel, 1987)

Phrases like 'pull yourself together', 'you shouldn't get involved', and 'if you think *you've* got a problem, just look at *my* workload' are heard far too often in nursing. And put up with.

The basis of assertiveness and of any management of yourself is **listening**: to yourself, to others, and to the environment. Only by listening do you actually hear what is happening. Without knowing what is going on you can't change anything; you are deaf. And how often we *are* deaf, or don't believe what we hear! When we don't hear and believe what others tell us about themselves, our deafness is a danger to their lives.

Stress

What exactly *is* **stress**? Selye (1976) says that it is 'a non-specific response of the body to any demand, whether it is caused by, or results in, pleasant or unpleasant conditions'.

Stress is non-specific; everyone reacts differently and has different signs. That is why stress is so difficult to pin down and why people who are experiencing it are so often not believed.

Dillon (1983) describes five stages of stress:

Stage 1: The honeymoon Stress challenges you.

Stage 2: Fuel shortage You have a vague sense of loss. Challenge and enthusiasm have waned. You experience job dissatisfaction, fatigue, sleep disturbances, and escape activities.

Stage 3: Chronic symptoms Physical illness and loss of control of your emotions are recognised by you and by others.

Stage 4: Crisis Your acid stomach becomes a bleeding ulcer. You become obsessed with your symptoms. Discontent becomes disillusion.

Stage 5: Hitting the wall You lose control of your life. Without help from others you may never regain that control.

It may be interesting to compare these stages with some of the topics discussed in this book:

- Stage 1 and Stage 2 have to do with motivation.
- Stage 3 could fit in with the non-assertive behaviours.
- Stage 4 and Stage 5 link in with the description of the people coming downstream, about to drown.
- Stage 5 may be the point where – with help – a person is able to discover the meaning of his or her life and return to the 'honeymoon stage' where life becomes challenging again. Sadly, that help is all too often lacking in nursing.

Stress is a necessary factor for survival, but where it leads to an excessive demand on an individual and beyond his or her ability to cope, stress becomes destructive. The result of too much stress is a person's total inability to function effectively.

In the early stages of stress the physical symptoms are the most obvious signs that something is amiss. Such signs are initially coping mechanisms:

- being tired and sleepy;
- overeating;

- drinking;
- heavy smoking;
- changing jobs;
- withdrawing.

(Albrecht, 1982)

- Do you recognise any of these signs in yourself?
- Are these signs there all the time or only at particular moments?

It has been said that reading and learning about stress *gives* you stress where before you had coped very well! On the other hand it may also give you insights into unrecognised aspects of stress, which can be helpful. Be aware of both possibilities.

With the physical signs go also the emotional aspects of stress:

- feeling useless;
- feeling incompetent;
- being touchy and irritable;
- having outbursts of anger;
- finding it hard to concentrate;
- weeping for no reason;
- experiencing violent mood swings;
- having feelings of panic;
- being unable to make decisions;
- being bored with oneself;
- having feelings of 'unreality';
- losing one's mind;
- becoming obsessive;
- having feelings of guilt;
- being impatient;
- having no more compassion;
- being insensitive to others.

Some people try to compensate for these feelings and work twice as hard, showing everybody that they *are* competent and *can* cope. In that way they feel less guilty. When this happens they really are on the treadmill. The sad fact is that only an outside source can stop it.

Debbie

Debbie had been ward sister of a small ward in a specialist hospital. The staff–patient ratio was high and the staff were of a high calibre. They needed to be, as in spite of excellent treatment regimes, many patients died on that ward.

Debbie was also a very pretty girl, but recently her make-up had become heavy and even grotesque. Over time the staff found her increasingly difficult to relate to. One of them complained that she had 'a heart of stone'. Various attempts were made to 'bring her to her senses'. Debbie did not see that there were any problems. She was not sick, worked hard – harder than most other ward sisters – and she got on well with the patients. She did not see that she didn't get on with the staff – not until she was suspended from duty.

Think of yourself here.

- Do you recognise any of these signs in yourself?
- How long have they been there?
- Do you recognise them in others?
- What do you do when you meet them in yourself and others?
- How often do you feel indispensable?
- Do you feel personally responsible for the destinies of others?

Remember the Gestalt 'prayer' (page 27).

Before looking at ways of dealing with stress it will be helpful to look more closely at the actual causes of stress.

Stressors

When you listen to yourself, to others, and to the environment, you realise that these three areas also form the three main sources of stress, or **stressors**.

Stress from the environment

The **nursing culture** as it exists in Britain has much to answer for in creating stress. The image of the 'handmaid' is disappearing, but slowly. The mere fact that so many nurses want to learn about assertiveness shows that they feel they are not coping.

The image of the nurse who always carries out orders and never asks 'Why?' is not such a caricature. A few years ago we were grappling with 'the unpopular patient': the patient who asked too many questions. We have had to accept that more and more patients these days do not simply say 'yes' and 'no' as appropriate. But nursing is having difficulty in accepting 'the unpopular nurse': the nurse who asks 'Why?'

Routine has been the hallmark of this culture. This was outlined clearly by Menzies (1960) in her well-known study. Routine and the status quo protected student nurses in particular from 'getting involved' and from stress. Or so it was thought. Menzies showed that on the contrary these *led* to stress: relationships once formed could not develop; work begun could not be followed through; and, most revealingly, taking no part in decision-making rendered nurses cold and uncaring. From the outline of the temperaments in Chapter 1 it can be seen that perceiving people tend to make good nurses: that is, people who do not care for routine, but who respond to the immediate surroundings.

- How much do *you* like routine?
- Does it help you, or stress you?
- Had you been aware that routine, deadlines, and doing things by the book might be stressors?
- Acknowledge any insights and be aware of the meaning they have for you.

If the hospital culture promotes stress, then so also does nurse education. The **pressure to succeed** (Farabaugh, 1984) is very strong. In the classroom it is easy to portray nursing in an idealistic light. And all around, the pressure is on for more qualifications and higher degrees. This pressure is necessary when looked at from the point of view of the work and its demands. When seen from the standpoint of individual nurses, though, the pressure may be too intense, and nurses need to be able to say 'no' and not feel guilty about it.

Nurses often experience **guilt** when their **expectations** of themselves and those put onto them by others do not match up. Learner nurses in particular will have learnt to make a bed in a set fashion, to take their time to talk with patients, and that they will never be let alone at first. Yet when they get to the ward, they find that beds are not made according to the book, that they have no time to talk with patients – or if they do they are told to 'do' something – and that they are left in charge when they have hardly learned how to *spell* 'haemorrhage'.

But not only the practical aspects cause stress. Nurses are required to give holistic care, be advocates of patients, leaders of teams, agents of change, responsible and accountable for their actions. Such ideals may not be achievable unless you know yourself well – your strengths and needs, your values and your boundaries, and where and when to enjoy yourself.

Work does tend to be the main stressor for people. But all sorts of environmental factors also cause stress:

- commuting to work;
- housing problems;
- visits to the dentist and hospital;
- constant noise;
- the lack of pleasant excitement;
- claustrophobic situations;
- emergencies and accidents.

You might like to add your own environmental stressors to this list and so become more aware of your surroundings and what they mean to you.

Stress caused by other people

To start again with the nursing culture, there is a strange *cruelty* pervading the profession. '*I* was thrown in at the deep end, so I make sure that I throw *you* in at the deep end'. The lack of support from superiors for subordinates is sadly endemic. It seems that what causes stress and burn-out most quickly is not hard work, rotten hours and low pay, but a *lack of positive enforcers*: of a 'thank you', of support, and of the chance to have the need for self-actualisation fulfilled.

Cook and Mandrillo (1982) found that 'workers who had the *responsibility for the destinies of others* were under greater occupational stress than were persons who were responsible for managing material assets'. 'Paper-pushing' may be stressful, but does not involve the whole person as much as does caring for others. It is usually the more sensing and feeling people who choose nursing, so it is not difficult to see that it is these very people who will suffer and get hurt in the process.

There has been a great deal of research into what stresses nurses most. A synthesis of some of them (Adey, 1987; Albrecht, 1982; Hingley & Harris, 1986; Seuntjens, 1982) appears below.

Look at the list, and add your own stressors, and perhaps number the items in order of your own priorities:

- work overload;
- staff shortage;
- death of a liked patient;
- unexplained changes;
- poor communication;
- lack of appreciation;
- lack of feedback;
- family difficulties;
- hardened attitudes;
- conflict of loyalties;
- breaking bad news;
- no say in policy-making;
- very ill patients;
- irregular work schedules;
- job responsibility;
- relationship with doctors;
- poor career prospects;
- role conflict;
- administrative hassles.

This list shows clearly that the majority of stressors for nurses do not arise in the work *per se*, but in the many *relationships* with other people involved with the work. Yet this is not so extraordinary, since most difficulties in life are caused by relationship difficulties. The problem of **conflicts of loyalties** cannot be overestimated. Too often nurses are 'piggy in the middle'. When it has been decided that a patient should not know his or her diagnosis it is the nurses who have the most delicate job; when a drug error has been made, it is the nurse who gets disciplined; when a policy is not carried out, it is the nurse who bears the brunt.

A positive move in the right direction is Clause 11 of the UKCC Code of Professional Conduct: 'Each nurse ... shall ... have regard to the workload of and pressures on professional colleagues and subordinates and take appropriate action if these are seen to be such as to constitute abuse of the individual practitioner and/or to jeopardise safe standards of practice'. Yet even this can turn sour, and a nurse who defends a colleague can easily be dismissed for meddling in affairs that do not concern her or him.

These phenomena are not peculiar to nursing: most people know similar types of stressors. What *is* peculiar to nursing is the lack of support and care. It is therefore not surprising that 'of all professional groups, nursing has one of the highest rates of suicide and nurses top the list of psychiatric outpatient referrals' (Hingley, 1984).

The stresses caused by and through other people in life generally tie up with those of work. It is not possible to separate life into 'home' and 'work' — indeed people who try to make them separate *add* to their stress, as in that way they split themselves into parts when everywhere else the trend is towards holism.

Bond and Kilty (1982) describe the stresses from other people as coming mainly from a *'bad atmosphere, inappropriate expectations or demands*, and *rejection*, or *not being understood'*. An awareness of other people and of their needs, and the ability to listen to them, will — or should — considerably reduce the stress created between people.

- What stressors act on you? Are other people responsible for these?
- What stressors act on others? Are you responsible for those?
- Are you aware of your needs?
- Are you aware of the needs of those who work with you?
- *When* are you most stressed?

Stress from within the self

There is much legitimate stress coming at us from outside ourselves over which we have no control. Simply the way in which life is lived and organised is stressful. But besides that, we ourselves put a lot of stress on ourselves, some of it willingly, some unwillingly; some quite unconsciously. The expression 'personal luggage' is a very apt metaphor for this aspect of life. Here are some of the issues which go into this luggage:

- expectations from childhood carried over into adulthood (and now acting as 'shadow');
- unresolved bereavements;
- guilt feelings;
- old resentments, now irrelevant;
- out-of-place ambitions;
- assumptions about others and oneself;
- perfectionism;
- not daring to succeed;
- feelings of dependence on others;
- not knowing when, where, or how to say no;
- inability to learn from mistakes;
- fear of illness, loss of control;
- a lack of confidence;
- fear caused by memories of life events;
- oversensitivity to ideas and influences;
- overcaring for others.

When looking at the meaning of a situation or relationship we may come across these things and they can block us. They each arrived there for a reason, but that reason no longer exists. Yet we still hang on to this luggage.

We cannot look at what stresses us without at some stage looking at these personal pieces of luggage. This fact brings us back to awareness, the temperament, the shadow, values, motivations, and ways of asserting ourselves. But it brings us back to these elements at a deeper level. To understand yourself at this level, you will probably need help.

As long as you were able to blame someone else — parents, the boss, the environment, 'they' — you were not responsible for your actions, nor for mistakes and failures from the past. When you look into yourself at the level of the stress produced from within yourself, you begin to see that the responsibility lies with you, and within you. But it takes a lot of personal strength to accept this, cope with it and use it positively.

Responsibility is a delicate issue. As we learn to take responsibility for ourselves and our actions, we learn also *not* to take responsibility for others. Many caring people have unclear boundaries, and therefore tend to 'take over'. They are the 'mother hen' types: the people with wide arms who can smother others. This, sadly, is not care for others, but care for oneself, or selfishness: it is stepping on other people's rights.

Learning to care and to be responsible means above all learning to be **empathic**: going alongside, caring, being a companion, giving **freedom**. A true responsibility grows out of freedom, and freedom leads to rightful responsibility.

But such insights and learning are almost impossible on one's own. As it concerns others, these things have to be learnt in company with others, and often in groups. Some of the means of support outlined in the next chapter may be of use to you. But before that, some more points about stress have to be addressed.

Coping with stress

There are as many strategies for coping with stress as there are reasons for stress or responses to stress. Overall there are two main approaches to dealing with stress:

- changing yourself and your attitudes;
- changing or removing the cause of stress.

Changing yourself

When you change yourself and your attitude you do not change the cause of the stress. But you do not allow it to hurt you any more. Another prayer may be appropriate here:

God grant me the serenity
to accept the things I cannot change;
courage to change the things I can;
and wisdom to know the difference.

Self-awareness does mean taking the time to sit down with yourself to listen to the parts of yourself that hurt, and are tense and stressed. There are many practical ways in which this awareness can be reached:

- relaxation;
- meditation;
- listening to music;
- chanting a mantra;
- praying;
- journal writing;
- imaginative drawing;
- visualisation/fantasy journeys;
- writing poetry.

One of the difficulties is that a stressed person usually has a short concentration span. And for any strategy to work, it has to be continued. To give up after one or two attempts is defeatist; miracles don't just happen: we have to work at them. It may therefore be helpful to do some of those exercises with the support of another person or a group.

Changing or removing the cause of stress

This is the real uphill work. The work you have already done on motivation and on assertiveness will form the basis of it, as will your values.

As a simple outline of the management of any change, the four steps of the Nursing Process form a good framework:

- assessment;
- planning;
- implementation;
- evaluation.

I have tended in this book to group topics under three headings. In each case the fourth would be **evaluation**. The various themes can be equated:

Assessment	Past	Memories	What is happening?
Planning	Present	Associations	What is the meaning of it?
Implementation	Future	Dreams	What are you doing about it?
Evaluation	Evaluation	Evaluation	Evaluation

Any strategy for change has to take into consideration what has gone before; what is the present reason for the change; and what is hoped for and expected from the change. Evaluation is not something that is tagged on at the end as an afterthought; it should go on throughout the process in the form of feedback and revision.

Valerie	Valerie had a difficult relationship with her mother. They saw each other about once a year only as her parents had moved to Scandinavia many years ago.
	Before going on her latest holiday, Valerie decided that being kind to her mother would be the best possible strategy and something that she could cope with. She would not allow an argument to develop, and instead of getting upset she would not allow herself to mind.
	Although they did have their differences, Val's decision meant that she did not get angry, and the inevitable contretemps did not poison the atmosphere. On her return she realised that she had actually *enjoyed* her holiday! Although this tactic did not solve the problem of the relationship, it made the atmosphere easier, and that was a good-enough goal for the present.

When you know your needs, wants and possibilities, you can begin to establish goals. When you know where you are heading to, you are free of the many unnecessary distractions that encumber your life and tend to drag you down. When you are working towards realistic goals you have become a round peg in a round hole, and have stopped trying to fit into someone else's (or your own) fabricated square.

Pot–Mees (1987) has outlined certain things that nurses should be and do in order to succeed without stress:

- be true to yourself;
- have realistic expectations;
- consider your own feelings as important.

Solving a problem under these circumstances may not seem as impossible as you had imagined! (The book *Managing Change* in this series will be of more detailed help on this point, and you are advised to read that for further help.)

Positive stress

One way of dealing with stress is actually to counter it with stress that gives you a 'high'. Here are some suggestions:

- competition/sport/physical activity;
- confronting difficulties directly;
- decorating a room;
- preparing and having a party;
- giving yourself a treat;
- doing something you would not normally do;
- giving yourself time out.

After having taken some practical – and possibly distracting – step, you may be able to face a particular problem in a new way, perhaps an unexpected way. You might also like to try the following exercise:

- Isolate your problem as clearly as you can. Then imagine that you are in the ideal world, without any constraints. You could be what you are, and do what you like best doing.
  - Where would you be?
  - What would you be doing?
  - Who would you be with?

- Take these questions seriously. Don't just *think* about them; let your imagination roam. Your fantasies are free – let them come and delight you.

- When you have in fantasy seen yourself without constraints, imagine now all the constraints that could possibly be put upon you.
  - What constraints are there upon you?
  - What constraints do you put upon yourself?

▶

Imagination is not simply kids' stuff. It is the greatest faculty we have for seeing possibilities. It is also, for adults, the single most under-used resource for moving forward. Trust your imagination, and use it to help you find your blind spots. When you have identified those, you are in a position to deal with them, and in this way move forward; when you can name something, you have a hold over it.

In my dream I had let myself be persuaded that I was needed in the disaster. I was following someone else's command without taking notice of my own needs, possibilities and feelings. Not being suited to that kind of work led me very quickly to become stressed, and unable to function effectively. Only when I took time out, looked inwards and outwards (and that with the help of a guide), could I realistically decide where my real place was: back on the ward.

I had to learn the hard way; this is part of my character and temperament. We all do it differently. What matters is that insight did come. The person who came to my aid believed in my stress, and so enabled this process to begin.

References

1 Adey, C. 1987. 'Stress: who cares?' *Nursing Times* **83**(4), pp. 52–3.
2 Albrecht, T. L. 1982. 'What job stress means for the staff nurse.' *Nursing Administration Quarterly* **7**(1), pp. 1–11.
3 Bond, M. and I. Kilty 1982. *Practical Methods of Dealing with Stress*. (Guildford University, Human Potential Research Project.)
4 Cook, C. B. and M. Mandrillo. 1982. 'Perceived stress and situational supports'. *Nursing Management* **13**(9), pp. 31–3.
5 Dillon, A. 1983. 'Reducing your stress.' *Nursing Life* **3**(3), pp. 17–24.
6 Farabaugh, N. 1984. 'Do nurse educators promote burnout?' *International Nursing Review* **31**(2), pp. 47, 48, 52.
7 Hingley, P. 1984. 'The human face of nursing.' *Nursing Mirror* **159**(21), pp. 19–22.
8 Hingley, P. and P. Harris 1986. 'Burn-out at senior level.' *Nursing Times* **82**(31), pp. 28–9.
9 McNeel, B. T. 1987. 'Stress.' In A. V. Campbell (ed.), *A Dictionary of Pastoral Care*. (London: SPCK, p. 268.)
10 Menzies, E. P. 1960. 'A case-study in the functioning of social systems as a defense against anxiety.' *Human Relations* **13**, pp. 95–121.
11 Pot-Mees, C. 1987. 'Beating the burn-out.' *Nursing Times* **83**(30), pp. 33–5.
12 Selye, H. 1976. *The Stress of Life* (2nd edn). (New York: McGraw-Hill, p. 74.)
13 Seuntjens, A. D. 1982. 'Burnout in nursing – what it is and how to prevent it.' *Nursing Administration Quarterly* **7**(1), pp. 12–19.

Chapter 6   Supporting yourself

Support

If I am not for myself
Who is for me;
and being for my own self
What am I?
If not now, when?

(Hillel 'the Elder', 70 BC–AD 10)

Support for nurses has long been declared an 'urgent top priority' (Briggs, 1972). But nothing much has happened to put this into practice. Sadly, more and more nurses are coming down the river about to drown.

Anne

Anne was a young sister on a surgical ward. Just before taking up her post, her father had died after a long illness. Her line manager, who had been very supportive, moved a few weeks later. Anne felt bereaved all over again. She began to have gastric upsets and was often 'scatterbrained'. Whereas before she could have joked about a mishap and coped, now she burst into tears. Her GP gave her a few days off; she dreaded going back to work. A friend suggested that they go together to a newly-formed women's group. There Anne began to realise that she was not alone with her feelings. The leader of the group suggested to Anne that she should also see a counsellor from CRUSE, the bereavement organisation, and gave her a name. Anne felt hesitant at first, but then took up the offer. After a few times of meeting she could understand her feelings and reactions better and was able to face the world again.

Support is many things. Each person needs different types of support, depending on temperament, work environment, and so on. Support is anything that:

- affirms you;
- encourages you;
- helps you to be creative;
- helps you to come to deeper insights about yourself and your life;
- helps you to fulfil your potential;
- helps you to have realistic goals in your life and keep working towards them;
- helps you to change goals, particularly during and after a time of crisis;
- challenges you.

> Stop for a moment and look at this list. Which area do you think is most applicable to you at the moment? Do you recognise anything of Anne within you? If you do, make a note of it.

In an ideal setting the employing authority would ensure that the necessary support was available to all staff. Employers have both a responsibility to their staff to see that they come to no harm (Hancock, 1983; Tschudin, 1985), and an interest in *keeping* staff, because experienced staff are valuable, and because turnover and absenteeism are very costly. All the same, neither self-interest nor legal requirements have as yet led many employers to provide adequate emotional support. If you want support, therefore, you have to go and get it. What you want badly enough, you will get. What is good enough to have is worth fighting for.

I have heard many a manager say, 'They can always come and talk to me', or, 'The occupational health department staff have counselling facilities', or 'If they want a group, they can have one'. This is cheap, and devaluing. In the area of support only the best is good enough. 'A chat' with the line manager is not always appropriate, and most OHDs are geared towards rehabilitation, advice and guidance, not professional counselling. And setting up an effective support group needs expertise and commitment.

In my dream a person came to give me support. That person was my own self, my 'shadow', that hidden part of my personality which I knew yet didn't know. Support is necessary to find and discover that 'person' within.

Five different possibilities of support will be outlined here. You may find that you need others as well. You may then have to go and get them. But keep in mind that what works for one person and one area may not work for another person or another area. You need to find the support that is appropriate for *you*.

Education and training

To achieve job satisfaction and prevent 'burn-out' and 'drop-out', a nurse must be self-directing and must maintain control over her own practice.

(Hickey, 1982)

This sums up quite neatly many of the things said in this book so far. One of the pillars of 'practice' is **training**. In nursing, post-basic training is often looked upon as a 'necessary evil', and is seen from a totally practical angle, such as training someone how to use some new equipment or for a specific role, such as management. But to give **job satisfaction**, nurses need more: they need **personal satisfaction**.

Education and training after registration should be very broad. In particular it should cover the aspects given below.

Interpersonal skills

- Interviewing skills
- Group/team leadership skills
- Supportive skills (particularly for and with dying patients and their relatives)
- Committee/chairmanship skills
- One-to-one helping and counselling skills
- Assertiveness skills
- Personal-defence skills
- Recognition and management of stress

Training and teaching in ethical issues

- Ethical principles
- The UKCC Code and its implications
- Issues such as advocacy, informed consent, accountability, confidentiality, responsibility

Management and assessment skills

- Management of a ward/unit
- Management of a budget
- Safety aspects
- Management of time and resources
- Assessment of learner nurses
- Assessment of auxiliary staff
- Assessment of volunteers

Have you had any training in any of these areas? Which, do you think, is the most important area in which you now need more training? Make a list of your priorities.

- Find the course you need (in the nursing press; through personnel officers; enquiring at training establishments, etc.).
- What is your *goal* in doing such a course?
- What do you *want* from such a course?
- What is your strategy when approaching your manager?
- How can you be working towards getting what *you* want, not what *he/she* wants from you?

▶

39

Mentors

In some hospitals, each nurse has a **mentor**. This person is not necessarily a friend, but one who has the overall well-being of this colleague in mind. The nurse concerned knows that there is one specific person to whom she or he can turn in the first instance.

A ward or unit organises itself in such a fashion that each nurse has one other nurse who is particularly responsible for her or him. They meet once a week for a conversation, even though they may also see each other every day. The mentor is first and foremost concerned for the physical well-being of the colleague, and checks that she or he is not overworked or underworked. If there are any specific difficulties, these can be discussed.

Co-counselling

Co-counselling is similar to mentorship but more structured, and its aim is wider.

Co-counselling is carried out in pairs, with each member possessing the same (or similar) skills and, furthermore, aware of the knowledge and skills possessed by the other. Additionally, co-counselling is organised by the two people so that each takes an *equal* amount of time to work as client and an *equal* amount of time to act as counsellor.
(Townsend and Linsley, 1980)

Basic training courses lasting about four days are available (contact the Human Potential Research Project, University of Surrey, Guildford GU2 5XH). The training consists mostly of techniques of 'undoing the "compulsive helper" habits and learning how to *assist* the co-counselling "client" rather than lead her' (Bond, 1986).

The basic premise of co-counselling is that many of our past hurts have been denied, hidden, repressed, or allowed to lie undiscovered. They have become outmoded luggage which we carry around with us to our detriment; or which do not allow us to realise our full potential. To deal with the memories, associations and dreams, and to find the potential and meaning of ourselves and of life: this is what co-counselling sets out to do.

On a practical level it needs two people who are willing to meet regularly and for a set and equal amount of time. It costs nothing (apart from the training), and the benefits are potentially enormous in terms of personal and professional satisfaction and success. Bond (1986) claims that nurses who co-counsel regularly 'feel better and seem to have less infections than before they took up co-counselling'. Under-used or unused skills can free a person. The benefits from the freedom can never be counted or analysed, only known and celebrated.

Counsellors

The definition of **counselling** of the British Association for Counselling is this: 'The task of counselling is to give the client an opportunity to explore, discover and clarify ways of living more satisfyingly and resourcefully.' All too often in nursing, 'counselling' is equated with disciplining. Because of that, nurses hesitate to make contact with a counsellor, or do not know what to expect if and when they meet one.

It is often a crisis, a point of recognition that 'I cannot cope any more', which brings a person to a counsellor. At such a time, however, it is impossible to think straight, feel clearly, get in touch with emotions and memories, or look to some future satisfying living. What the person (client) needs is to be heard, to feel accepted and not judged, and to be given support in whatever way is appropriate to cope with the next few hours or days. Only after that can the real work of counselling and development begin.

The concept of this book, managing yourself, is precisely what counselling is about: to enable you to get to know yourself, your strengths and needs, to find motives for your values, to find meaning and potential for living, and to have the ability to put this into practice.

In a counselling situation, the presenting problem is very often not what eventually turns out to be the main focus. The main focus is the *person*, your way of being and doing, and this can occasionally take quite some time to come to terms with. The strengths and needs, the temperament and the shadow are often reluctant to reveal themselves.

Because each person is so different, it is almost impossible to say either what goes on in counselling, or what counselling should be or could help you with. The more aware you are of yourself, your strengths, your needs and your failings, the easier counselling might be — or the more demanding and challenging.

If you are looking for a counsellor or a counselling service, you should always assure yourself of certain points:

● Is it *professional*? Is the counsellor trained, and how well? Many people who have done a two-day course call themselves counsellors; this is deceptive and can be dangerous.
● Is it *confidential*? Is no one going to know about your visits unless *you* tell them?
● Is it *independent*? To whom is the counsellor accountable? (This is why counselling services in OHDs and schools of nursing must be somewhat suspect.)

It has been said that counselling is 'for better or for worse'. A counsellor can be an effective 'midwife', so that the client can solve his or her own problems, form his or her own goals, and adjust his or her style of living. But an ineffective counsellor may not be able to handle such situations well.

Much *helping* is done quite incidentally in daily life: it is often invaluable and quite adequate. This, however, is not counselling, though it may make use of some of the *skills* of counselling.

Support groups

Support groups are perennial discussion points because of their regular appearance and disappearance. Nurses want to set them up, but then do not have the knowhow or the incentive to keep them going.

Support groups will only be effective if they are action-orientated. They should 'deal with issues of professional identity; with techniques for stress management; methods of conflict management; increasing staff members' sense of self-esteem and self-confidence, while increasing their knowledge and skills in nurse–patient interactions' (Scully, 1981).

Within such a framework support groups are very variable. They may:

● have one goal;
● have several goals;
● meet weekly;
● meet monthly;
● have a leader;
● take turns at leadership;
● meet for a set number of occasions;
● be on-going;
● be for nurses only;
● be interdisciplinary;
● be for nurses of one grade only;
● be for all staff on a unit/ward;
● be a time for relaxation and sharing;
● have a fixed agenda;
● be small;
● be large.

The main reason why groups are often difficult to maintain is the lack of a goal. One of the most important — and least often asked — questions is, 'What is your purpose?' or 'What is your aim?' Nurses are always quick to find solutions, and a support group may be a 'solution' to a particular situation, but the problem may not have been analysed and the purpose of it may not have been sought. In the first enthusiasm the group will 'work' for a few times, but then it will simply fizzle out — unless it has a purpose or objective, and unless that purpose is clear to all participants and can and will be regularly evaluated by them.

How are you supporting yourself?

Throughout this book I have been asking you to be aware of yourself, your thoughts, feelings, motives and needs, and to note them down. This was done to enable you to gather your energies and focus them in an exercise to help you manage yourself more effectively — more resourcefully and more satisfyingly.

The quote at the beginning of this chapter —

If I am not for myself
Who is for me;
and being for my own self
What am I?
If not now, when?

— could be an ideal starting point for a personal philosophy, an 'aims and objectives' for your life, or for writing your personal set of principles.

If you want to get anywhere you have to have a plan, a strategy. You need to know the how, who, where, what and why of a thing or situation before you can be a part of it, or tackle it.

Much of life is a constant striving for control. Humankind's survival depends on the individual's ability to master the environment. This is not so much a domination of others ('I am the boss around here') as a co-operation with and adaptation to the given situation. This takes effort, and the stress produced in the process is considerable — unless you know what you can and what you can't do, and what the difference is.

As a part of what this book can give you, I would like to invite you therefore to work out your personal philosophy and to make that a part — even the basis — of the way in which you manage yourself. The following questions and exercises are suggestions in formulating such a philosophy. If you have better, or other, questions and means, then please do use them.

What is good in your life at this time?
● Make a list and find as many things as possible.

What is difficult in your life at present?
● Make a list of the items you recognise, or refer to your notes of earlier exercises.

What do you recognise as weak or undeveloped characteristics?

What do you recognise as particular needs?

What life events have formed you most?
● In what ways? Be as specific as you can.
● What has changed for you after such (an) event(s)?

Who are you when you are alone?

What three things about your life do you value most?
● If you could have just one value, which one would you choose?
● Study your motives for choosing this one, and note it down.

What do you like most about your colleagues? your friends? your family?
● What do you think they like most about you?

What do you like *least* about them?
● You cannot change them, you can only change yourself and your attitudes to them. What change might you want or need to make?

What meaning is there for you in the relationship with a close person (name the person)?

What meaning is there for you in the relationship with a person (name him or her) with whom you do not get on but with whom you cannot avoid contact?

What motives keep you wanting to help other people?
● Do you help them, or do you help yourself?
● Empathy is said to be the ability to get close to a person, but keeping one foot on firm ground in order to help that person objectively. What is your firm ground in helping?

▶

When things go wrong, do you blame *them* (the things) or *someone*? Do you blame yourself?
- How much responsibility do you take yourself in unfortunate circumstances?

Do you recognise any particular needs that you have at the moment, but have not yet mentioned?
- Think about them, then note them down.
- Check with the diagram on page 26 to see in which category your needs are. Are they all in one, or in different categories? What do you deduce from this about yourself?

One person's personal philosophy statement runs like this:

I am I.
I am responsible for myself.
When I feel myself responsible for others I take away their freedom.
When they take away my freedom, I am diminished.
Therefore I have to say no, not defiantly, but creatively, for myself and to them.
When I am lonely I tend to use others for my own ends.
When I know my firm ground it gives me comfort, strength and joy. Only I can cultivate my own ground.
Others are my friends in so far as I am a friend to them. I cannot expect them to give of themselves. When they do, it is beautiful.
I can will, and strive, and yet I may not succeed. Having done all, and not succeeded, I will accept what is given, and not regret.
When I know my limits of strength, courage, empathy, and go as far as those limits but not beyond them, I am wise.
Wisdom teaches me to extend my limits ever wider in patience, goodness, and respect. I can and will accept the challenge.

(Mäder, 1988; translated and adapted)

This is how one person has formulated the main ideas of the meaning of her life. She felt it necessary to make it clear to herself that she has the responsibility for her own actions. She is helping herself in order to help others. This example may give you some hints about the kind of things you would like to say about yourself.

The last two points in the statement quoted may sound contradictory. This is deliberate. A statement of philosophy is a guide, a map, an indicator of the limit or boundary of yourself and your world. But you are not 'bound' by such a document. Self-awareness has a 'growing edge', and from time to time the statement has to be rewritten, and adapted. It is not a tablet of stone.

Supporting yourself is looking after yourself. When you know your self, your strengths and needs, then you are comfortable with yourself — comfortable enough to go beyond yourself and help and care for others in such a way that they are enhanced, not dominated; freed to be creative themselves, not dependent. This is why support is so important: it helps you to become yourself; and through that others become themselves.

References

1 Bond, M. 1986. *Stress and Self-Awareness: a guide for nurses.* (London: Heinemann, pp. 100, 104, 173, 213.)
2 Briggs Report, 1972. *Report of the Committee on Nursing.* (London: HMSO.)
3 Hancock, C. 1983. 'The need for support.' *Nursing Times*, **79**(38), pp. 43–5.
4 Hickey, J. V. 1982. 'Combating "burn-out" by developing a theoretical framework.' *Journal of Neurosurgical Nursing*, **14**(22), pp. 103–7.
5 Mäder, D. 1988. (Personal communication.)
6 Scully, R. 1981. 'Staff support groups: helping nurses to help themselves.' *Journal of Nursing Administration* **11**(3) pp. 48–51.
7 Townsend, I. and W. Linsley 1980. 'Creating a climate for carers.' *Nursing Times* **76**, pp. 1188–90.
8 Tschudin, V. 1985. *Ethics and Management of Support for Nursing Staff.* (North East London Polytechnic: unpublished B.Sc. (Hons) dissertation.)

Chapter 7　　　　　Celebrating yourself

Celebrating

He who is able to celebrate life can prevent the temptation to search for clean joy or clean sorrow. Life is not wrapped in cellophane and protected against all infections.

(Nouwen, 1978)

By celebrating I don't mean sitting back and letting the world go by. As awareness exists only in order to go beyond it, so **celebrating** yourself means celebrating yourself *and* celebrating the other person. How, you may ask, does this relate to managing yourself?

Self-awareness comes into its own when awareness of others is authentic, liberating and creative. You manage yourself well in relation to others; you manage others well in so far as you manage yourself well. This means finding a balance between work and play, personal and professional life.

The three elements of past, present and future which I have used repeatedly can also be applied to celebration. I would like to start with the present, with affirming, before going on to look at the other elements of celebrating, namely remembering and expecting.

Affirming

Celebrating is **affirming** yourself and affirming life. But like awareness, this is not easy to do these days for two reasons.

Firstly, celebrating means taking time. But the world is in a hurry: a sense of breathlessness pervades all we do. An advert is only valid if it states that the job is for this 'busy' ward or centre. A meal is not a time for rest and company, but a mere stop for refuelling. Always rushing about means never affirming anything. Always looking for more and better, means simply getting there faster. But where?

Secondly, the opposite is also true: those who do not rush about stay asleep. These are the armies who cannot be bothered, who find anything an effort. They give you the impression that one day they will not even know the difference between a wedding and a funeral.

Either by rushing about, or by being asleep, we have largely forgotten how to celebrate. We generally celebrate only good things; by bringing 'bad' things into awareness we 'celebrate' them also. Staying with the good and the bad for a while gives us insight. Because we don't celebrate the 'bad' things we don't learn from them. We put up heroes and leaders and imagine that their qualities will do the work for us.

As a first step in affirming yourself, stop and think:

- Who are the three people, living or dead, who you admire most? Write down their names.
- Who are your heroes? Write down their names.
- What are the qualities for which you admire them?

When you have thought about that, try to recognise those same qualities in yourself.

Affirming yourself gives you confidence and satisfaction and the ability to evaluate yourself. When you know yourself, your strengths and your needs, then you are less tempted to seek approval from others – approval which might well be only flattery anyway.

When you know who you are or what you are, you do not need to wear a mask, or look for status or authority. When you know yourself and are sure of it, you are an **authentic** person. Then you can say with all simplicity, 'that is what I do best, and that is what gives me satisfaction'.

Self-awareness and self-knowledge give you a **freedom** to be yourself and express yourself in appropriate and easy ways. Freedom is the real reason for this celebration.

But maintaining that sense of affirmation and freedom is not easy. **Power** and **authority** can creep up surreptitiously, and selfishness then abuses that power. This is why celebrating is not an ego-trip. It is done in order to become more authentic, more real, more open.

When you are affirmed – by yourself and by others – then you can affirm others.

It is usually in moments of crisis, doubt or failure that someone needs to be affirmed most. When you have failed in some way – real or imaginary – you don't need to be told, 'serves you right'. You need to have someone there who asks, 'What happened? Tell me, I'm here to listen.' When you know what it felt like for you, you have a good idea what it may feel like for others. You can make use of your experience, both of the crisis and the resolution of it, to help others. This is **empathy**. Being there does not mean taking over. The difference between effective and ineffective help lies here: giving attention gives the other room to grow; taking over is a selfish act. Affirming is respecting the person, and respecting his or her freedom; taking over is abusing this freedom.

Rogers (1975) has described empathy as being not only a skill, but 'a very special way of being'. Roach (1984, see page 14 of this book) described compassion as 'a way of living'. 'Getting involved' with another is inevitable; in fact it is the only possibility. This is when the boundaries become unclear and the edges blurred. But in doing that each recognises the humanity of the other. They are not helper and helped any more, but each helps the other. That is when the edges begin to 'grow'.

Respecting the other also means not judging that person, nor any way of life, action, situation or view until you have heard the story about it. It is so easy to make assumptions, to jump to conclusions, to finish a sentence for the other. That is taking over and assuming a responsibility which we have not been given. We affirm others only when we hear *their* story. Respecting the other helps him or her to grow and be creative. In respecting, you are respected. In creating, you are created. Some people have called this **co-creativeness** – an apt term for this kind of work.

When this stage is well established, the next step is that of **being supportive**. It is not an imposing stance, but a 'being-alongside' as the person finds his or her own way.

People don't like to be 'should' upon. They'd rather discover than be told.

(Dass & Gorman, 1985)

When we 'should' on others, we take away their freedom. Another person's freedom is her or his basic right. When we take it away, we diminish our own freedom.

Supporting is helping others in every way to complete their work of creating. It may mean challenging them to wake up, or challenging them to slow down. Whatever it is, it is a being-alongside while they find *their* goal, *their* purpose – of life, themselves, their actions.

That can only be done with a great deal of **hopefulness**. Those who prefer to sleep tend to be afraid of the future; those who rush about have no sense of the past. The truth lies in the middle, in the present. To come to that middle, that authentic way of being, is hard work, with many trials and failures. If we believe that another person is worthy to be affirmed, then we need the hope to support her or him not just to a goal, but on the path to that goal.

Remembering

When there is no **memory**, there is nothing to celebrate. We can only stand in the present because of the past where we have come from.

The reason for rushing about is often to forget, to eradicate, and to make-believe it never happened.

Other people give their memories power to destroy them. In the film *The life that's left*, a family is shown in which one of the young sons had been killed in an accident. His mother kept his room just as he had left it. The other members of the family were not to laugh any more in the house. There was literally a deathly hush all over the house. The memories were gradually destroying the family as a whole, and the individuals in it.

Memories are 'the stuff of life'. To live life to the full we have to *hear* our own and other people's memories.

... most people here [in the nursing home] ... they just want to tell their story. That's what they have to give, don't you see? And it's a precious thing to them. It's their life they want to give. You'd think people would understand what it means to us ... to give our lives in a story.

So we listen to each other. Most of what goes on here is people listening to each other's stories. People who work here consider that to be ... filling time. If only they knew. If *they'd* just take a minute to listen!

(Dass & Gorman, 1985)

We each have our story to tell. Before that, we each have our story to *make*. We are responsible in large part for what we do with our lives and ourselves.

- If you were to write your autobiography, what highlights – which memories – would you choose for an outline?
- Choose any one particular memory and stay with it. Is it a good memory or a difficult one? Simply be aware of it and of your choice: don't judge it.
- In what way has this memory shaped your present – that is, in what way are you still celebrating this memory?

Memories are important aspects of our lives. **Traditions** in families and nations keep a wider memory alive for the future. Religions keep sacred memories and memorials and celebrate them regularly. In order to be what we are we have to realise where we have come from.

The best things in life – family, friends, health, nature – come free, and therefore we are inclined to think that we have a right to them. Yet they are not ours to *keep*, but to *treasure*. To take them for granted is to overlook their intrinsic worth.

Celebrating by remembering is 'counting the blessings', seeing the good, the noteworthy and the advantages.

On page 20 I asked what keeps you in nursing. The answer you gave then is relevant here: celebrating the memory shapes your present, and your future.

Give yourself permission to celebrate your successes. Such celebration is the basis of your professional confidence.

Our celebrating of memories allows us to help others celebrate theirs. Self-awareness is fulfilled when it leads to helping others come to new insights, new celebrations.

When you have been with a person and affirmed her or him, there comes a time when you need to look inwards. In order to discover the *meaning* of a situation, an event, or life, you need to see it in the perspectives of your memories. Has anything like this happened before? What was the outcome? What does this remind you of? The memories then lead to associations with the present, and that is the raw material for finding a goal to move forward.

Paul	Paul was an elderly patient on a medical ward. On the day the consultant came, Paul suffered violent diarrhoea which could not be explained. An observant staff nurse noticed that when Paul complained of diarrhoea again it was again the day of the consultant's visit. At an opportune moment the nurse tentatively enquired about the diarrhoea. She soon found out that Paul's father had 'died of diarrhoea'. Paul's father had been a patriarch of the first order, and the consultant looked uncannily like him. After a while it became evident that Paul was terrified of dying because that was when he would be meeting his father again.

Memories from the past suddenly come into focus. Associations are made which to an outsider might not make much sense, but which to the person concerned are (literally) of *vital* importance.

When these memories are brought into the present, acknowledged, 'counted' one by one, and given the attention necessary, then the whole person is affirmed.

Expecting

We can look back only because we have a sense of the future. It may seem a contradiction in terms to say that we need to celebrate the future. Only in the dictionary does success come before work. . . .

We celebrate the future by creating it.

Neither the sleepers nor the rushers have much of a sense of the future. Without a sense of where you are going you are not getting anywhere. This is why it is so important to have goals, or meaning, in life; without them people drift here and there – physically and emotionally.

Throughout the reading of this book, you have looked at yourself. In thinking about your own meaning and your own philosophy of life you have prepared the way for celebrating your future. The next chapter should help you to put this into practice.

When you have experienced the need for some goal, meaning or direction in life, then you can also help others to come to similar insights.

- What are you expecting from your life?
- What do you hope it will give you?
- What are you prepared to give to life?

By celebrating what you expect, you are also celebrating those as yet unknown or undeveloped parts of yourself: the shadow. The shadow is part of you, longing to be acknowledged. Some parts of it will always remain hidden, but the areas that have been revealed in and through the memories and associations ask to be taken seriously and dealt with. This is indeed where celebrating the expectations comes in: by not being afraid and thereby restricting the future. **Fear** inhibits so much growth. Celebrating the future is a kind of celebrating of the abandonment of fear.

Discovering a meaning in life, setting yourself a goal, or describing your purpose, often opens up a wide vista. To come to an insight, exclaiming 'I see', is really to see into the future. It is like a huge leap forward. It is that essential step from the present unsatisfactory mode to the future and more satisfactory way of being.

Alice and Dick

Alice and Dick were in their late fifties. They had not been able to have children and had suffered all their lives. As their nieces and nephews grew up, they took a lively interest in *their* families. They were godparents of Annabel and helped with great interest to organise her wedding. When a few years later Annabel told them that she and James could not have children either, the two couples sat for a long time together, crying and being aware of their pain and what this had meant for each. It was James, Annabel's husband, who said finally, 'You've helped me understand what suffering is about.' This seemed quite incredible to Alice and Dick, who had only felt pain. They looked at each other and tears started again. But this time they were tears of joy. Annabel and James had given them the gift of themselves, and beyond their pain they seemed to be falling in love all over again. They could have no children, but they had each other to cherish. Their old age suddenly seemed like a new life.

- Do you remember the last time when you had an *aha!* experience? How did it happen? What has changed for you?
- Stay with the experience as you remember it, and see how it has brought you forward. Have you taken it for granted, or are you grateful for it? How?

To stand with another person at the point of expecting the future, 'dreaming' about it and seeing possibilities, is to be present at one of the most exciting moments that life can offer. I have talked in terms of helping someone; in truth it is not so much 'helping' someone else as enabling another to become what she or he already is. You are not so much a helper as a 'midwife' to an experience. In that role you are not only helping another: you are fulfilled yourself.

Rogers (1978) describes well what this means:

I have found my greatest reward in being able to say 'I made it possible for this person to be and achieve something he could not have been or achieved before'. In short I gain a great deal of satisfaction in being a facilitator of becoming.

You might like to think – remember – a similar time or experience when you have been with someone, perhaps agonising for a long time before coming to a conclusion, a goal, a decision, or an insight. When that moment came, the other was helped, but you were affirmed in your own person too.
● What was the turning point?
● What memories do you have of it?
● In what way can these memories now help you? In what way are you, or should you be, celebrating them?

'Celebrating' in an authentic way is going back to awareness, and seeing it as from a new angle. *Awareness* is looking at yourself from 'outside'; *celebrating* is looking at yourself from 'inside', from experience. Awareness is knowing what 'strokes' you give to others, and they give to you, and how and when you give and get them. Celebrating is living them; but they are not simply strokes any more: empathy – sharing – has become a way of life.

This is what managing yourself is about: being with others in such a way that both you and they are freed, liberated, moved forward. When you manage yourself you celebrate yourself, and those around you.

In the dream I had to stand in the rubble for a long time; become a part of it, even. I had to remember a great deal and make it my own – to celebrate it. Only in doing that, in not escaping but hearing the rubble around me speak and becoming aware of the rubble, the suffering within me too, could I finally feel 'me' again.

We are made up of ruins which have been made for us and which we have made for ourselves. But ruins need not rule our lives. They invite us to go beyond them, into the future, to acknowledge their potential and to believe in it. *That* is celebration.

References

1 Dass, Ram and P. Gorman 1985. *How can I help?* (London: Rider, pp. 157, 112–13.)
2 Nouwen, H. J. M. 1978. *Creative Ministry*. (New York: Image Books, p. 95.)
3 Roach, M. S. 1984. *Caring: the Human Mode of Being, Implications for Nursing*. Perspectives in Caring Monograph 1. (Toronto: University of Toronto.)
4 Rogers, C. 1975. 'Empathic: an unappreciated way of being.' *Counselling Psychologist* **21**, pp. 95–103.)
5 Rogers, C. 1978. *On Personal Power*. (London: Constable, p. 92.)

Chapter 8   Your career – making the choices   *by Jane Schober*

When you qualify in your chosen field of nursing you face an ever-increasing number of work and career opportunities. At the time of qualifying your choices may be influenced by the availability of posts, by pressures on you to gain certain experience, and by expectations from your school of nursing about what constitutes suitable experience. Nevertheless, the choices you make early in your career are just as important as those made later on. An initial qualification is the first step, but if you wish to progress not only clinically but in other areas (such as nursing management, nursing research and nursing education), further study is usually required, and many posts now demand extra qualifications. This chapter suggests approaches that may help you make effective career moves and career choices.

Now more than ever before, all nurses need to consider seriously the implications of choosing not only certain *posts* within the profession, but also particular courses of *study*, whether these relate to clinical nursing (for example, National Board clinical courses), management (for example, staff-nurse development courses and ward-sister courses), or education (for example, courses which lead to registration as a nurse tutor). There is a marked relationship between the quality of your work experiences, the pursuit of your career, and your personal and professional development. You therefore need to identify what motivates you at work (see Chapter 3), the social and personal factors that affect your work (see Chapter 1), and those things that contribute to your job satisfaction.

It is perhaps especially pertinent to explore these issues now, at a time when various changes in nursing are directly affecting careers at all levels. These changes concern the education of nurses, with the introduction of Project 2000 and the clinical grading structure; and the problems associated with staff shortages, such as increased workload, stresses at work, and, in some areas, low morale. Many of these issues result in uncertainty for nurses already in post who are being expected to adapt and develop their roles to accommodate the changes. Faced with these changes you need to identify your sources of **support, guidance** and **resources**, and thereby win access to relevant information and the time and opportunity for learning and personal development. If you take time now to explore what a career may hold, and the benefits to be gained from *planning* a career, you will discover ways of improving the short- and long-term decision-making relating to your career.

To plan and pursue a career encourages you to develop personally and professionally. This in turn increases job satisfaction, improves work choices, and promotes overall progress. However, studies have shown that, within the UK, although the idea of a career in nursing is well recognised – and indeed favoured – by society, surprisingly little **career guidance** is available to registered nurses (Schober, 1987; Schober, 1988).

What is a career?

Explanations and meanings of 'career' include such definitions as:

Course or progress through life, way of making a livelihood for advancing oneself, personal advancement and success in life.

(Oxford English Dictionary, 1979)

The references here to success, progress and advancement suggest that a career can result in the experience of personal satisfaction and that a career can be very much a part of one's life. As such, it should be highly valued.

Other commentaries take this further. Van Maanen and Schein (1977) suggest that there is both an *'internal' career*, a career which is personal and part of one's own perception, and an *'external' career*, which has characteristics that are recognised by society or by the members of a particular occupational group. They define an internal career as:

A set of steps that make up the individual's concept for the progression within an occupation.

and the external career as:

The more or less objective categories used by members of society or of an occupation to describe the typical or official progression of steps through a given occupation.

These definitions of a career highlight the importance of your personal perception of work and occupational experiences (as outlined in the definition of an internal career), and also the influence that society, or the expectations of a particular occupational group, may have on you as an individual member of that group. You need to consider the place of these two approaches to what a career may mean, and to try to regard a career from both points of view when considering personal work choices.

This is particularly true if you remain in a given role for several years. Other members of the organisation, for example your managers or colleagues, may after a while suggest that it would be in your interests to consider a change or promotion. (This not uncommonly happens after only two years in a more senior role.) You may experience conflict if you are quite content to remain in your role for much longer than is generally regarded as the norm; to change at a time when **job satisfaction, learning** and **motivation** all exist within your role *may* lead to disillusionment and dissatisfaction. Moreover, you yourself may be more aware than others of your own limitations, and you may consider the stress of moving on more than you wish to cope with; or you may, rightly or wrongly, be suspicious of your manager's motives for encouraging you to move. Career guidance in situations like this can help to reduce the potential conflict faced by an individual vulnerable to the pressures of other people's expectations.

Other definitions of career deserve examination. Rapoport and Rapoport (1980) suggest that a career is:

A sequence of occupational jobs which were developmental in character and which required a continuous and high degree of commitment.

This reference to **commitment** is a characteristic that has been recognised as important to effective nursing (Altschul, 1979). Here may be seen a relationship between purposeful practice and the importance of a well-chosen **career path**. If it is true that your career is closely related to developments within your job (as indicated in this definition), it follows that you yourself should be involved in the decision-making about your occupational choices, and that you should be helped to recognise how such choices are affecting your personal and professional development.

Table 8.1 gives five meanings of 'career'.

Table 8.1 Characteristics of a nursing career

(1)	A successful professional life
(2)	Advancing or developing a role
(3)	Membership of a profession
(4)	A lifelong sequence of jobs
(5)	A sequence for role experiences

(Hall, 1976)

Hall (1976) suggests that career development is part of being a professional. If so, effective decision-making about career choices is also part of being a professional, and therefore your own responsibility as much as your employer's (though the organisation for which you work may be able to offer guidance).

Hall's reference to success suggests that your career choices will lead to positive outcomes and therefore to personal satisfaction. To make this more likely, it is important to consider how you may gain **feedback** from those around you (particularly from your managers): feedback helps you to recognise how effective your performance is within a given work role, and thus within the organisation. Remember, though, that 'success' in this context may look different from the managers' and subordinates' perspectives.

Making career decisions

Very few nurses or employees of the Health Service have recognised responsibility for career guidance. Often nurse tutors are looked to for advice and guidance, particularly by nurse learners and newly-qualified staff. It has been shown also that registered and enrolled nurses seek advice from nurse tutors who work within departments of continuing education (Schober, 1988), with whom they have regular contact.

Other possible sources of career guidance include the advice that may be obtained through **performance appraisal** interviewing. Many such systems consider the career needs of the individual. Such planned appraisals afford an excellent opportunity for managers and subordinates to discuss ideas and expectations relating to job satisfaction, performance potential, educational needs, and short- and long-term career choices. However, studies in the UK suggest that the provision of such appraisal is limited.

In developing your career — important as this is as a part of your life — it is vital that the choices you make are made with as much information, support and guidance as possible.

You need to begin by considering the management of your life in *all* its aspects: effective career decision-making must take into account the whole of your life — not just your work or career needs, but also your family, social, and personal needs. Morrison and Zabelman (1982) suggest that successful career-committed nurses have just this wide understanding of their needs.

Start by identifying aspects of work, family and personal needs which are important to you: these may determine whether certain changes in role are wise. See Table 8.2.

Table 8.2   Personal factors affecting career choices

Work needs	Personal needs	Family/social needs
Job satisfaction	Job security	Partner's continuing support
Promotion	Salary	
Increase in responsibility	Status of the role	Availability of child care
Need to work	Enjoyment of the role	Availability of accommodation
Interest in the work	Familiarity within the organisation	Travelling distance from home
Hours of work		
Motivation to learn	Reluctance to change roles	House prices
		Family's need of the income

Table 8.2 simply highlights *some* of the factors you need to consider. Identify which of these are important for you, add to the list any others that will help you when you come to assess the suitability of a post.

Try always to be clear about the factors that contribute to your job satisfaction. First reflect on previous nursing experiences, for example those in clinical posts. Reflect on aspects of your clinical nursing experience both while a learner and since registration. Try to describe the aspects of previous experiences that you liked the best and those that you liked least. Then try to explain to yourself why this was. Tables 8.3 and 8.4 offer some prompts which may help you.

Reflect on these factors and add to the list others that are relevant to you. You should be able to identify factors which cause you to enjoy aspects of work; factors which motivate you and provide you with the incentive to go on learning within that area; and factors which give you a sense of satisfaction because of your contribution to the work process within that area.

Table 8.3 Factors influencing job satisfaction in a clinical post

- Factors relating to care
- The clinical specialty
- Mixed or unisex wards
- Pace of work
- Nurse–patient relationship
- Involvement in technical aspects of care
- Teaching patients
- Counselling of patients and relatives
- Surgical aspects of care
- Medical aspects of care
- Rehabilitation
- Health promotion

Table 8.4 Professional aspects of the experienced nurse's role

- Being a member of a multi-disciplinary team
- Being a member of a nursing team
- Being a primary nurse
- Being a team leader
- Being in charge
- Teaching other nurses
- Assessing other nurses
- Night duty

Personal goal-setting

Now try to identify **personal goals** which will help you to make appropriate decisions about your career. The following goals are guidelines which may help this process.

Self-knowledge

Use **self-knowledge** of factors previously mentioned, together with feedback from managers and those with whom you work, to clarify the skills and qualities that you possess in the workplace.

Information retrieval

Gather **information** relating to areas of interest, courses of study, new workplaces, and new posts.

Education and training

Be aware of **educational and training opportunities** both locally and nationally. You should be able to get summaries of courses put on by your local department of continuing nurse education, your district training centre, your regional training centre, local and national colleges, polytechnics and universities. You should also find out about opportunities offered by your professional organisation (for example the Royal College of Nursing, the Royal College of Midwives, the Health Visitor Association or the District Nurses Association).

Advertisements

Study any **advertisements** for posts which may interest you. Look in the local and national press and in the nursing press. Consider advertisements for nursing, midwifery, management, nurse education and posts outside the National Health Service. Gather facts about each prospective post, including details of status, grading, length of contract, role, opportunities for ongoing professional development, and terms and conditions of service.

Curriculum vitae

Formulate a **curriculum vitae** (CV). Guidelines for this are given in Table 8.5. A CV is an important, and ideally an impressive, summary of personal and professional details, and is usually complementary to a completed application form. An up-to-date CV is a particularly important feature of the application for any senior post.

Table 8.5   A suggested layout for a curriculum vitae

Name		
Address	Date of birth	Age
General education		
Professional qualifications		
Professional education		
Present appointment		
Previous appointments		
Research		
Publication		
Professional interests		
Referees		

Mentors

Take advantage of a **mentor** if possible (see Chapter 6). It has been found that those who work closely with a mentor benefit greatly from the personal and professional advice and guidance. Hardy (1986) found that in general male nurses take advantage of this far more than do female nurses, which may be a factor contributing to the number of male nurses in senior posts.

Referees

Choose **referees**. These people are essentially your backers when you apply for a particular post. Referees are not bound to disclose to you what they have said, and indeed should not be asked to do so. It is essential that they feel able to be absolutely honest in their appraisal of you, and this may be impossible if they are asked to give details. You should, therefore, choose carefully whom you ask to give a reference.

Remember always to keep your referees informed of the details of your applications for posts and courses. It is likely that you will want to use them on more than one occasion, so it is important that you not only notify them of the outcome of applications but express your gratitude, as appropriate, for their support.

The ultimate decision about your career pattern rests with you. You are the only person who can weigh up the professional, personal and social factors that affect your own life and find a working balance between them all.

To **know yourself** – your limitations as well as your potential – should be the rule.

Planning your career — the choices

Following **registration** or **enrolment**, the choices facing you are many and varied. Initially you need either to gain experience within the health authority where you have trained or to look for some other post in which you can gain experience as a newly-qualified nurse. Thereafter, the main choices are as follows:

(1) nursing in a hospital setting;
(2) nursing in a community setting;
(3) undertaking a further course of statutory training;
(4) undertaking a programme of continuing education;
(5) joining the Armed Forces;
(6) nursing overseas;
(7) nursing in the independent sector.

There are other careers which might benefit from the discipline of a nursing training — for example government service or research writing.

Nursing in a hospital setting

On entering a part of the register or roll by completing a course of **statutory training**, be it RGN, RMN, RNMH, RSCN, RM or EN, initial posts are likely to be in a hospital setting or — in the case of those registering as RMNs or RNMHs — in a unit closely allied to the hospital.

Within each of these specialties there is a vast range of job choices: it is usual for nurses to choose whenever possible to gain further **experience** in a ward, unit or department where they have had some experience as a learner. This allows you to consolidate your previous knowledge and to develop skills relating to clinical management, personal skills, counselling skills, teaching skills and decision-making skills, which previously will not have been possible. For many, this first post following registration or enrolment will offer the longest period of allocation to one particular area. It is usually helpful at this stage to stay in one role for at last six months, so that you can develop more confidence and skills in the area.

A wide range of posts is available to registered and enrolled nurses within a hospital setting. They are summarised in Table 8.6.

Table 8.6   Clinical nursing posts available in a hospital setting

- Nursing adults needing surgery
- Nursing adults with medical problems
- Nursing adults with a mental illness
- Nursing adults with a mental handicap
- Nursing women, and midwifery care
- Nursing children
- Nursing the short-stay patient/client
- Nursing the long-stay patient/client
- Nursing the acutely ill
- Nursing the chronically ill
- Nursing the dying

There is a similarly wide range of roles and specialist posts available for registered nurses. A broad selection of these may be found in Table 8.7.

Table 8.7   Examples of nursing posts in a hospital setting

- Staff nurse, e.g. ward, unit, clinics, out-patients
- Ward sister
- Night sister

▶

Table 8.7 continued

- Midwife

- Clinical nurse specialist, e.g. intensive care, behavioural therapy

- Stoma nurse

- Infection-control nurse

- Diabetic liaison nurse

- Continence advisor

- Research nurse

- In-service training sister

- Nurse manager

- Nurse teacher/tutor

Continuing education opportunities

Departments of continuing nurse education have developed and flourished, over the past ten years in particular. These departments have a two-fold function: first, to provide opportunities for **in-service education** for registered and enrolled nurses, and training and support for nursing auxiliaries and support workers; secondly, to set up and run **clinical courses** for the English National Board (or other National Board, as appropriate). These range in length from six weeks to one year, depending on the intentions of the course and the specialty. The ENB approves these courses, and there now exist specialist clinical courses relating to most fields of clinical practice for RGN, RMN, RNMH, RM, HV and DN (see Table 8.8).

Table 8.8   Summary of the main ENB courses for registered general nurses

- Accident and emergency nursing

- Anaesthetic nursing

- Burns and plastic-surgery nursing

- Continuing care of the dying patient and family

- Coronary care

- Dermatological nursing

- General intensive care

- Neuromedical and neurosurgical nursing

- Nursing elderly people

- Oncological nursing

- Operating department nursing

- Orthopaedic nursing

- Paediatric medical and surgical cardio-thoracic nursing

- Psycho-sexual counselling

- Special and intensive nursing care of the newborn

- Stoma care nursing

- Renal and urological nursing

- Rheumatic disease nursing

- Sexually-transmitted diseases

Many other **specialist courses** are available for registered mental and mental-handicap nurses – the ENB will supply a complete list on request.

On completion of these courses the National Board issues either a statement of attendance, for courses lasting between 5 and 30 days, or a certificate, for the longer courses which last between six months and one year. ENB courses exist for registered and for enrolled nurses. For many specialties there exists a course for both enrolled *and* registered nurses. Information – about the duration of these courses, the centres and schools of nursing which run them, and the outlines for each course – may be obtained from the ENB Resource and Careers Service in Sheffield.

Many of these courses are extremely popular. The National Boards generally recommend that before applying for a place on one of the longer courses you should have been qualified for between six months and one year. It is also worth checking with a chosen centre to see whether there are any additional criteria for entry to such a course – for example some centres may look for previous experience in a specialist area.

Other courses validated by the National Boards include **short courses** relating to developments in and aspects of nursing care, for example in general nursing, mental-illness nursing or mental-handicap nursing. There are also courses that orientate qualified nurses to aspects of professional development, for example research appreciation, and teaching and assessing in clinical areas. These courses are open to registered nurses, and are particularly useful for those who wish to develop skills which will allow them to contribute to the quality of clinical care, through study and application of theory and knowledge associated with these areas. For nurses wishing to obtain senior clinical posts, these courses are particularly helpful; they have been shown to be relevant to those who supervise both basic and post-basic learners, those who are assessors and mentors in a clinical area, and those who are involved in clinical developments.

Alongside opportunities which exist in most schools of nursing for the pursuit of a specialist clinical course, there are also courses run by departments of continuing education which provide **in-service education and training** for nurses at *all* levels. Many of these departments offer a current programme of in-service education for staff nurses and ward sisters. Though some of these courses are compulsory for these groups within the health authority, the fact that they are co-ordinated plans of study which run concurrently with increasing clinical responsibility allows those on the course to continue to learn while gaining knowledge and experience of new roles.

In the light of the clinical grading structure, you now need as a clinical nurse to be aware of any **educational requirement** associated with a post. The advent of longer in-service programmes for registered nurses reflects the vast development that has taken place in post-registration nurse education. It is a significant development from earlier training opportunities. Examples include **study days** associated with updating nurses in clinical practice and in changes in policies and procedures.

Opportunities for hospital-based enrolled nurses The cessation of enrolled nurse training has led to the introduction (and increasing number) of **conversion courses** for enrolled nurses. Demand for these places is great, with many enrolled nurses facing delay and perhaps disappointment in their pursuit of a place on such a course. If this is your position, take advantage of other opportunities to enhance your practice and your own personal and professional development. Some ENB **clinical courses** are open to enrolled nurses and there are also in-service educational opportunities. Nursing leaders are looking at ways of adapting educational programmes for enrolled nurses so that these nurses may be able later to use an ENB clinical course towards their ultimate registration – 'distance learning' is one possibility.

Opportunities for registered nurses The introduction of Project 2000 heralds major developments in the theoretical content that will accompany nurses' clinical experience in the future. Over the past ten years in particular growing numbers of nurses have pursued courses of further study to develop a greater knowledge base and a broader theoretical framework about nursing, behavioural sciences, social sciences, education and management. The University of London **Diploma in Nursing** has been, and still is, a popular choice amongst registered nurses who wish to pursue **part-time courses** which offer opportunities to study psychology, physiology, sociology, nursing theory and nursing research, as these relate to their own clinical areas. Courses are available all over the country. Most are based in polytechnics and colleges of higher education. Also, the Distance Learning Centre at the South Bank Polytechnic in London is now offering this course to those who do not have easy access to a college. (Details of the Diploma in Nursing may be obtained from the Department of Extra-Mural Studies, London University.)

Other areas of significant growth are the number of **degree** courses open to nurses. These include degrees in nursing, health studies, psychology, education and physiology, and degrees by research. (Details of Bachelors' and Masters' degrees for nurses may be obtained from the ENB Resource and Careers Service in Sheffield.)

Nursing in the community

Educational opportunities for those who choose to work in a community setting are also varied. Existing roles are summarised in Table 8.9.

Table 8.9   Roles for nurses within the community

- District nursing

- Health visiting

- School nursing

- Practice nursing

- Community psychiatric nursing

- Community mental-handicap nursing

At the present time there are courses of study available to qualified nurses which lead to each of the qualifications and roles identified in Table 8.9. However, work has begun in looking at how the education of nurses who work away from a hospital setting may be made more effective. One idea, for example, is to merge district nurse training with the training of health visitors (Baker, 1988).

District nursing

Courses are available for both registered and enrolled nurses which may lead to the appropriate **District Nursing Certificate**. Following the DN Certificate and after appropriate experience, nurses may apply for training to become practical-work teachers. This involves the education and training of district nurse students and subsequently opportunities for career progression to more senior educational posts.

Health visiting

The pursuit of a career in health visiting demands that you be a registered nurse, and that you have midwifery experience and an academic background which includes at least five GCSEs. There are also some universities that run **degree** courses for nursing which contain a health visiting option. Health visitor training and education is based in colleges of further and higher education; courses last one year, full-time. Following two years' experience as a health visitor it is possible to undertake further training to become a fieldwork teacher and to take responsibility for the practical training of student health visitors.

School nursing

School nurses need to be qualified as an RGN or a Registered Sick Children's Nurse (RSCN). Education is usually available in colleges which are already running health visitor courses. The school nurse is a member of the primary health-care team and plays a significant part in the health assessment and health education and promotion of children at school.

Practice nursing

Practice nurses are based in general practitioners' surgeries and carry out nursing duties. GPs may or may not require that the practice nurse has qualifications additional to RGN.

There has been much discussion about the nature of the practice nurse's role. Ample opportunities exist for nurses to extend their role alongside that of the general practitioner: indeed, many practice nurses undertake such activities as immunisation, suturing, patient assessment and health education.

Community psychiatric nursing

Over recent years, with the closure of large mental hospitals, there has been an increase in the number of mentally-ill people being cared for in smaller units, for example houses and hostels, under the close supervision of experienced nurses with RMN qualifications. The **Community Psychiatric Nursing** course is now available at a large number of centres. The course lasts nine months.

Further details of the course and a list of centres can be obtained from the ENB Resource and Careers Service in Sheffield.

Community mental-handicap nursing

Following the achievement of the statutory **Registered Nurse Mental Handicap** (RNMH) qualification, nurses may also pursue the **Community Mental-Handicap** course (nine months' duration).

A number of new educational opportunities exist for nurses working in therapeutic communities. These courses are particularly useful for community mental-handicap nurses and community psychiatric nurses, and are open to registered nurses with appropriate experience. All these courses are run at the Institute of Advanced Nursing Education (IANE). The **Certificate of Therapeutic Community Practice** course is open not only to nurses but also to social workers, occupational therapists and other members of the health-care team. The course lasts for one year, part-time.

Holders of the Certificate of Therapeutic Community Practice are then eligible to take the **Diploma in Community Mental-Health Nursing** and **Diploma in Therapeutic Community Practice**. These courses are run over one academic year and include a programme of tutorials and seminars, and a submission of a dissertation. Experienced community psychiatric nurses are eligible for this course if they hold the ENB Community Psychiatric Nursing Course 810 and 811 qualifications and have a minimum of two years' community psychiatric nursing experience.

For further information and details, contact the IANE, Royal College of Nursing, London.

Education for midwives

Following statutory education to register as a midwife (RM), you may take a number of ENB **clinical courses**. They include special and intensive care of the new-born, a 26-week course. There are also a number of **short courses** – see Table 8.10.

Table 8.10   ENB short courses available to registered midwives and registered nurses

(1)   Family-planning nursing
(2)   Short course on special and intensive nursing care of the new-born
(3)   Short course on the care and rehabilitation of physically-disabled people
(4)   Short course on diabetic nursing
(5)   Short course on the care of the dying patient and his/her family
(6)   The continuing care of the dying patient and the family*
(7)   Short course on the principles of psycho-sexual counselling*
(8)   Introduction to the understanding of the application of research
(9)   Teaching and assessing in clinical practice

*These courses are also open to enrolled nurses.

For further details of all these courses, and lists of centres which run them, contact the ENB Resource and Careers Service in Sheffield.

To pursue a career in midwifery teaching it is necessary to complete the **Advanced Diploma in Midwifery** (ADM). These courses are either full- or part-time and are run in schools of midwifery and colleges of further or higher education.

Nursing management

Entry into a nursing management post from a clinical post demands much of the individual nurse, not least that she or he is able to adapt to, respond to, and come to terms with, the different priorities in such a role.

Historically the education and training available for nurse managers has been extremely limited, but in recent years, particularly since the Griffiths recommendations were made, there have been several key developments in the provision of **management training**. The National Health Service Training Authority (NHSTA) has concentrated much of its activity on the development and provision of management training for all managers within the Health Service. Opportunities for nurses usually exist at regional training centres and in many health authorities at district training centres, where short and long management and administration courses are held.

All nurses are managers, many having extensive managerial responsibilities from the time when they become staff nurses and are involved in the management of a ward, a staff of nurses, and of patients and visitors. For nurses who wish to pursue more formal education in aspects of management, a number of opportunities exist. The first step is to look closely at the provision of management courses by departments of continuing nurse education in schools of nursing. **Staff-nurse development courses** and **ward-sister courses** provide excellent opportunities for nurses to begin to identify their wider management potential and the personal attributes relevant to effective management, and are vital for the promotion of professional development.

Within many colleges of further and higher education, **certificate, diploma** and **degree** courses relating to management are offered. The **Certificate in Management Studies** (CMS) is a useful course for junior managers as it introduces them to the principles of management, professional issues and organisational and personnel management. The IANE at the Royal College of Nursing offers a Certificate in Management Studies, which is a part-time course covering one academic year, for those at ward-sister level and above. From this course candidates may then go on to the **Diploma in Health Services Management**, which covers a further academic year and aims to extend management knowledge and skills for more senior and general management decisions.

Nurse education

Nurse tutor preparation

Developments in nursing education have led to teaching becoming an integral part of the role of most registered nurses. For clinical nurses interested in developing teaching skills, the ENB Course 998, **Teaching and Assessing in Clinical Practice**, is an extremely useful, though rather short, introduction to aspects of teaching, learning and assessing.

For those interested in formalising their teaching role a little further, the City and Guilds Course 730 in **Teaching**, which again is a part-time course over a period of six months, is a useful way of developing classroom and practical teaching skills. However, neither of these two courses offers nurses a recordable teaching qualification with the UKCC.

Until 1988 there were two recordable qualifications for nurse teachers. They could either follow a course to become a clinical teacher, which usually took six months' full-time study, or they could pursue a course of study which led to a qualification. Today you need to take a course that leads to registration as a **nurse tutor**. Suitable courses are summarised in Table 8.11.

Table 8.11 Courses that lead to nurse tutor registration

(1) Certificate of Education

(2) Diploma in Education

(3) Diploma in Nursing Education

(4) Bachelor of Arts in Nursing Education (Manchester University)

(5) Bachelor of Education

Certificate of Education and **Bachelor of Education** courses are available in many universities and colleges all over the country. The **Diploma in Nursing Education** course is a University of London diploma which is run at the Institute of Advanced Nursing Education, the Royal College of Nursing, London. The **Bachelor of Arts in Nursing Education** (Manchester) is also run at the Institute of Advanced Nursing Education and at Manchester University. This is a modular degree programme which has been developed with particular emphasis on nursing education.

Entry to these courses is determined by the National Boards. All nurse teachers must be first-level nurses. They must possess at least three years' full-time nursing experience within the past seven years, at least two of which must have been at staff-nurse level or above, in an area approved for training by a National Board. Evidence of post-registration study is also necessary. The Director of Nursing Education within the health authority sanctions applicants for nurse tutor courses. The National Board funds these course places and pays the salaries; certain expenses are also covered, for example a grant is made towards the purchase of books.

A full list of centres offering courses that lead to registration as a nurse tutor may be obtained from the Institute of Advanced Nursing Education, the Royal College of Nursing, London, and from the ENB Resource and Careers Service in Sheffield.

Teaching district nursing and health visiting

To become a district nurse teacher or a health visitor teacher you need to have at least two years' experience as a qualified district nurse or health visitor immediately prior to undertaking the course. These courses are held in universities or institutes of further education, and run for a year, full-time.

Teaching midwifery

To become a midwife teacher you need the **Advanced Diploma in Midwifery** and to have worked as a midwife for a year immediately preceding the course. The teaching course lasts one year, full-time, at a university or college of further education.

For lists of centres running all the courses mentioned here, contact the ENB. Resource and Careers Services, Sheffield.

Conclusion

While there remains a general lack of career guidance for nurses, it is important that you seek and use advice to make the best possible decisions relating to your career.

Your decisions must take into account the essential elements in all parts of your life. If you wish to work for most or all of your possible working life, if you are the essential breadwinner in your family, or if you choose to work around family commitments either in a full- or part-time capacity, job satisfaction and feeling good at work will ultimately determine the quality of your personal and professional development as well as your motivation at work. Such things as increases in salary, promotion and successfully completed courses are important contributors to job satisfaction, but they tend to be temporary, the reward from them often being short-lived, and other factors may outweigh the positive effects of these. Recognising this helps you to identify personal feelings of frustration, dissatisfaction, unhappiness and stress.

Such feelings are useful indicators that all is not well: they are prompts to take stock of the situation in which you find yourself.

There are formal and informal ways of identifying positive and negative aspects of your working life. Formal systems which help to clarify such issues include **performance appraisal, interviewing, staff groups**, and **problem-solving groups**. Informal ways include informal **meetings** and **discussions** with subordinates, managers, and peers. **Friends** at work and **social groups** contribute to this process.

Effective career decision-making depends on personal insights, on the understanding of the factors that motivate you at work, on the availability of career information, advice and guidance, and on feedback about personal and professional expertise and performance at work. By recognising and acting on these needs, you can do much to influence your own future as a member of the caring service.

Sources of career information

Directory of First Degrees and Diplomas of Higher Education (annual). (London: Council for National Academic Awards (CNAA).)

ENB publications relating to ENB course syllabuses, names and addresses of centres and details of ENB courses, statutory courses of training, occupational health nurse training courses, nurse teacher courses, first and higher degree courses for nurses. (Sheffield: English National Board.)

Directory of Schools of Medicine and Nursing (annual). (London: Kogan Page.)

Hospitals and Health Services Yearbook (annual). (London: Institute of Health Services Management.)

Institute of Advanced Nursing Education (IANE) prospectus (long and short courses). (London: Royal College of Nursing.)

Directory of Nursing Scholarships, Bursaries and Grants. (London: Royal College of Nursing.)

Useful addresses

Central Register Clearing House Limited
c/o English National Board
Victory House
170 Tottenham Court Road
London W1P 0HA

Council for National Academic Awards
344–345 Grays Inn Road
London WC1 8PT
Telephone: 01-278 3718

Distance Learning Centre
South Bank Polytechnic
P.O. Box 310
London SW4 9RZ
Telephone: 01-228 2015

District Nursing Association
57 Lower Belgrave Street
London SW1W 0LR
Telephone: 01-730 0110

English National Board Resource and Careers Services
P.O. Box 356
Sheffield S8 0SJ
Telephone: 0742 551064

Health Visitors Association
36 Eccleston Square
London SW1V 1PF
Telephone: 01-834 9523

Institute of Health Services Management
75 Portland Place
London W1N 4AN
Telephone: 01-580 5041

Institute of Personnel Management
35 Camp Road
London SW19 4UX
Telephone: 01-946 9100

National Board for Nursing, Midwifery and Health Visiting for Northern Ireland
RAC House
79 Chichester Street
Belfast BT1 4JE
Telephone: 0223 238152

National Board for Nursing, Midwifery and Health Visiting for Scotland
22 Queen Street
Edinburgh EH2 1JX
Telephone: 031-226 7371

National Health Service Training Authority
St Bartholomew's Course
18 Christmas Street
Bristol BS1 5BT
Telephone: 0272 291029

Northern Ireland Health and Social Services Training Board
The Beeches
Hampton Park
Belfast BT7 3JN
Telephone: 0232 644811

Open University
Walton Hall
Milton Keynes
MK7 6AA

Royal College of Nursing
20 Cavendish Square
London W1M 0AB
For courses: Institute of Advanced Nursing Education
For advice about working abroad: International Department
Telephone: 01-409 3333

Royal College of Nursing (Northern Ireland Board)
17 Windsor Avenue
Belfast BT9 6EE
Telephone: 0232 668236

Royal College of Nursing (Welsh Board)
Ty Maeth
King George V Drive East
Cardiff CF4 4XZ
Telephone: 0222 751373

Royal College of Nursing (Scottish Board)
44 Heriot Row
Edinburgh EH3 6EV
Telephone: 031-225 7231

Royal College of Midwives
15 Mansfield Street
London W1M 0BE
Telephone: 01-580 6523

Universities Central Council on Administration
P.O. Box 28
Cheltenham
Gloucestershire GL50 1HY

University of London
Department of Extra-Mural Studies
26 Russell Square
London WC1B 5DQ
Telephone: 01-636 8000

Welsh National Board for Nursing, Midwifery and Health Visiting
Floor 13
Pearl Assurance House
Greyfriars Road
Cardiff CF1 3AG
Telephone: 0222 395535

References

1 Altschul, A. 1979. 'Commitment to nursing' (The Battersea Memorial Lecture 1978). *Journal of Advanced Nursing* **4**(2) March, pp. 123–5.
2 Baker, J. 1988. *What next? Post-Basic Opportunities for Nurses.* (Basingstoke: Macmillan Education.)
3 Hall, D. T. 1976. *Careers in organisation.* (London: Goodyear, p. 4.)
4 Hardy, L. K. 1986. 'Career politics: the case of career histories of selected leading female and male nurses in England and Scotland.' R. White (ed.), *Political Issues in Nursing*, Vol. 2, pp. 69–82. (Chichester: Wiley.)
5 Morrison R. and E. Zabelman 1982. 'Tie career concept in nursing.' *Nursing Administration Quarterly*, Fall, pp. 60–8.
6 *Oxford English Dictionary* 1979. (Oxford: Clarendon Press.)
7 Rapoport, R. and R. N. Rapoport 1980. 'Three generations of dual career family research'. F. Pepitone-Rockwell (ed.), *Dual Career Couples.* (Sage, p. 23.)
8 Schober, J. E. 1987. 'Lighting the way.' *Nursing Times & Nursing Mirror* **83**, 9 Dec, pp. 66–7.
9 Schober, J. E. 1988. *Tie Career Guidance Experiences of Registered Nurses.* (Cardiff University: unpublished MN thesis, available in the Steinberg Collection, the Library, Royal College of Nursing.)
10 Van Maanan, J. and E. H. Schein 1977. 'Career development'. J. R. Hackman and J. L. Suttle (eds.), *Improving Life at Work: Behavioural Science Approaches to Organisational Change.* (London: Goodyear, pp. 30–95.)

Index

revision 36
rights 24, 27, 29, 34, 45
routine 32

satisfaction
  job 39, 40, 44
  personal 39, 40
school nursing 57
self-actualisation 26, 33
self-advocacy 16
self-awareness 3, 6, 17, 43, 45
self-confidence 41
self-discovery 3
self-esteem 41
self-knowledge 5, 45, 52
self-respect 19
senses 4
'sensing' people 6, 8, 21
shadow 8, 34, 39, 41, 47
short courses 56, 58
skills 39, 52, 54
  of assessment 39
  of counselling 41, 54
  interpersonal 39
  management 39, 54
  personal 54
  teaching 54
speciality 52
spontaneity 7
staff nurse development 59
strategies 42
strengths 32, 41, 43

stress 30, 34, 61
  causes of 35
  occupational 33
stressors 32
study days 56
submissive behaviour 23
success 40, 51
  pressure 32
suicide 33
support 38, 45, 49, 51
support groups 41

teaching 56
  skills 59
Teaching and Assessing in Clinical
    Practice 59
temperament 5, 7, 10, 32, 34, 38, 41
'thinking' people 6, 8
traditions 46
training 39
trust 29

values 10, 13, 17, 21, 27, 32, 41
  attitudinal 10, 13
  creative 10, 13
  experiential 10, 13
  nursing 14
  personal 13
  professional 13
visualisation 35

wants 24, 27, 29
ward sister development 59
workload 33